Surgical Essentials of Immediate Implant Dentistry

Surgical Essentials of Immediate Implant Dentistry

Jay R. Beagle, DDS, MSD
Private Practice
Indianapolis, IN

WILEY-BLACKWELL

A John Wiley & Sons, Inc., Publication

This edition first published 2013 © 2013 by John Wiley & Sons, Inc

Wiley-Blackwell is an imprint of John Wiley & Sons, formed by the merger of Wiley's global Scientific, Technical and Medical business with Blackwell Publishing.

Editorial Offices
2121 State Avenue, Ames, Iowa 50014-8300, USA
The Atrium, Southern Gate, Chichester, West Sussex, PO19 8SQ, UK
9600 Garsington Road, Oxford, OX4 2DQ, UK

For details of our global editorial offices, for customer services and for information about how to apply for permission to reuse the copyright material in this book please see our website at www.wiley.com/wiley-blackwell.

Library of Congress Cataloging-in-Publication Data

Beagle, Jay R.
  Surgical essentials of immediate implant dentistry / Jay R. Beagle, DDS, MSD, private practice, Indianapolis, IN.
    pages   cm
  Includes bibliographical references and index.
  ISBN 978-0-8138-1606-7 (hardback : alk. paper) – ISBN 978-1-118-51757-4 (epub) – ISBN 978-1-118-51760-4 (emobi) –
ISBN 978-1-118-51761-1 (epdf/ebook)   1. Dental emergencies–Handbooks, manuals, etc.   2. Dental implants.   I. Title.
  RK305.B37 2013
  617.6026–dc23

                                        2012039433

A catalogue record for this book is available from the British Library.

Wiley also publishes its books in a variety of electronic formats. Some content that appears in print may not be available in electronic books.

Cover design by Jen Miller

Set in 9.5/12pt Palatino by SPi Publisher Services, Pondicherry, India
Printed and bound in Singapore by Markono Print Media Pte Ltd

1   2013

I dedicate this book to my daughter, Jenna, who kindly allowed me a significant amount of father–daughter time to complete this text.

Contents

There is no question that endosseous dental implants have revolutionized tooth replacement therapies. Credit goes to Dr. P. I. Brånemark for his observation that optical titanium chambers integrated into the bone tissue and were difficult to remove. Since that time and his experiences in the oral edentulous cavity, many techniques have developed depending on the specific indications one encounters as patients present with missing teeth. This includes replacing a single tooth, short spans of partially edentulous spaces where several teeth have been lost, or replacing the entire dentition in an arch. Dr. Andre Schroeder expanded the biological implications of tooth replacement by showing that the dental implant could be placed into the bone and extend into the oral cavity at the same time, similar to the natural dentition. This option provided the groundwork for another variation in the dental implant technique, namely the immediate replacement of a tooth when it is removed from its alveolar housing.

The technique for the immediate replacement of the tooth, however, has proven to be a challenging technical exercise due to the various aspects that must be considered when replacing the root with an immediate endosseous implant. It is fortunate that Dr. Jay R. Beagle has taken his considerable expertise and time to share how this technique can be accomplished in a predictable manner. Dr. Beagle is a highly successful and extremely well-respected private practitioner who has many years of experience in dental implant therapy. Colleagues from around the world have sought Dr. Beagle's advice and learned from him as he has lectured worldwide. Perhaps most uniquely, Dr. Beagle has a keen sense of the scientific literature and puts into practice scientific methodology as he publishes clinically relevant papers in the field of dental implantology. He is also a major contributor and respected Fellow of the International Team for Implantology (ITI) and participates actively at the national and international levels. It is through these experiences and his many years of running a highly successful periodontal practice that Dr. Beagle brings us this comprehensive book on the immediate surgical placement of endosseous dental implants.

The contents of this book take the reader through all aspects of the clinical considerations for the immediate replacement of a tooth root with an implant. Most importantly, Dr. Beagle has supported each aspect with considerable scientific references. The advantage to the reader comes in the fact that by applying the science with Dr. Beagle's respected clinical skills and experience, you gain the knowledge required to accomplish this complex technique in a predictable fashion. The significance of predictability in this crucial implant indication is the basis of this comprehensive review and is achieved by Dr. Beagle based on his success in a large referral practice and his helping thousands of patients over many years of private specialty clinical practice experience.

Many aspects of replacing a long-time missing tooth where large amounts of native bone have filled in the socket are routine and can be accomplished by following a dental manufacturer's standard instructions. This is not, however, the case when one chooses to replace the tooth immediately after the root is removed, due to the fact that the precise surgical drill placement becomes not only difficult due to the lack of bone, but the angulation of the handpiece and bur must also be exact in spite of their being only open space where the root(s) used to be. Adding to the complexity is the often frequent need to place the tip of the drill onto the side of the socket wall and begin the drilling sequence on a steep vertical incline. Because the essence of esthetic and pleasing tooth replacement is the precise position of the implant, the immediate surgical placement of the implant in an extraction site is a complex procedure with risks. Dr. Beagle is careful to point out how this procedure must be thoroughly evaluated and all aspects of placement considered with all risks comprehensively reviewed, considered, and communicated to the patient.

In the introductory chapter, Dr. Beagle explains the historical development in the scientific literature for the immediate surgical placement of an implant into an extraction socket and explains that this technique can be predictably successful; however, many factors must be taken into account, and in every respect, the clinician must be evidence-based in

his or her technique. In chapter 2, Dr. Beagle's mantra for his outstandingly successful career comes out by stating that your goal as a clinician is to provide the best care for your patient while at the same time subjecting him or her to the least risk or complication. Dr. Beagle helps you achieve such a goal by providing you his knowledge and expertise in this area gained over his extensive reading of the literature and years in practice. Perhaps the greatest challenge in this particular technique and, in fact, all of dentistry is making your decisions as to when and how to apply any technique. This chapter is essential to the reader so that every patient and every tooth is exhaustively evaluated so that any pitfalls can be prevented. In chapters 3 and 4, Dr. Beagle provides helpful hints to more precisely evaluate the specific potential site for implant placement. Inherent in this discussion and a sign of Dr. Beagle's considerable clinical expertise are not only the indications for the surgical considerations of immediately placing an implant into a tooth extraction socket but also the contraindications. Both wise and experienced, Dr. Beagle is clever to point out that this technically challenging procedure is not always indicated, and a smart decision can be to not perform this procedure. Guiding the reader to help make that decision is what Dr. Beagle does in these two chapters.

Chapters 5, 6, and 7 are where Dr. Beagle uses his considerable clinical expertise to describe surgical techniques for removing the tooth root while minimizing socket wall trauma and to discuss how the immediate implant is carefully placed into an acceptable and ideal position. He also uses experimental data from the literature to explain how the extraction socket will heal, undergoing three-dimensional architectural changes. In the last chapter, Dr. Beagle acknowledges that like all procedures performed in patients, complications do and will occur. His vast experience and knowledge in this area is evidenced by his comprehensive review of the potential complications and his discussion (again highly evidence-based) of how they are managed.

In summary, Dr. Jay Beagle has written an extraordinary and comprehensive clinically relevant and evidence-based book on the surgical placement of dental implants into the sockets of immediately removed teeth. Dr. Beagle has carefully reviewed all aspects of this challenging technique and has well articulated the risks, treatment planning, techniques, and possible outcomes of such therapy. It is an easy read with interspersed pearls of wisdom and important and essential aspects to consider. Dr. Beagle provides helpful hints and reminders so that once read, the book will continue to be helpful as a reference manual. Because Dr. Beagle is comprehensive and scientifically evidence-based in describing this technique, the reader is much more assured of an excellent patient outcome—a goal we all desire. Dr. Beagle has applied the literature to the clinical technique rather than just stating evidence, thus going well beyond what is done in most books.

The amount of time and degree of preparation for this book by Dr. Beagle is obvious from his detailed literature support for his statements. That combined with his years of clinical practice make this an important contribution to anyone with an interest in dental implants. Dr. Beagle provides the reader with a clear and concise summary of experimental studies and evidence, but the book is written in such a straightforward fashion, it does not interfere with his clinical descriptions, which makes it a clinician's dream. It is my privilege to congratulate Dr. Beagle on an outstanding contribution to the field of dental implantology. There is no doubt that this book will serve as a landmark reference for those interested in the surgical placement of an endosseous dental implant into the socket of an immediately extracted tooth.

David L. Cochran, DDS, MS, PhD, MMSc

Acknowledgments

I wish to acknowledge my restorative colleagues in Indiana, without whose friendship, professional collaboration, and trust in allowing me to participate in their patients' care none of this would have been possible; my staff, for their daily hard work and superb patient care; John Walters, for his tireless and cheerful assistance in preparing this text; and finally, my wife, Patti, and my daughter, Jenna, for their unwavering love and support.

Introduction

The initial report in the literature regarding the placement of an implant immediately following tooth extraction was published by Schulte in 1976 (Schulte and Heimke 1976). It was not until the early 1990s that the concept was reintroduced in the English-language literature by Lazzara, who illustrated this method of treatment with three case reports (Lazzara 1989). Lazzara's landmark paper provided insight into the future of surgical implant dentistry, with technical aspects that remain critical today. The immediate placement treatment protocol was validated in the literature several years later by Gelb, who reported on a series of fifty consecutive cases followed over a 3-year period, providing a survival rate of 98% (Gelb 1993). Since then, numerous animal studies, human case reports, and several randomized controlled studies have furthered the science of this treatment modality (Figures 1.1–1.3) (Chen, Wilson, et al. 2004; Chen, Beagle, et al. 2009).

An understanding of the clinical and histologic realities of bone resorption that naturally occur following tooth extraction originally led to the concept of placing implants into sockets immediately following tooth extraction. This concept attempted, and still attempts today, to take advantage of the pre-treatment alveolar ridge contours (Chen, Wilson, et al. 2004). Many have noted additional advantages of this technique including reduced treatment visits and costs, simplified restorative care, and improved patient psychological outlook for treatment (Lazzara 1989; Parel and Triplett 1990; Shanaman 1992; Werbitt and Goldberg 1992; Denissen, Kalk, et al. 1993; Schultz 1993; Watzek, Haider, et al. 1995; Missika, Abbou, et al. 1997).

Numerous published works now indicate that outcomes of immediate placement procedures can be equally successful as a delayed approach when initial primary stability is achieved (Barzilay 1993; Schwartz-Arad and Chaushu 1997; Mayfield 1999; Chen, Wilson, et al. 2004; Chen, Beagle, et al. 2009).

The intent of this book is to provide clinicians with essential evidence-based information

Surgical Essentials of Immediate Implant Dentistry, First Edition. Jay R. Beagle.
© 2013 John Wiley & Sons, Inc. Published 2013 by John Wiley & Sons, Inc.

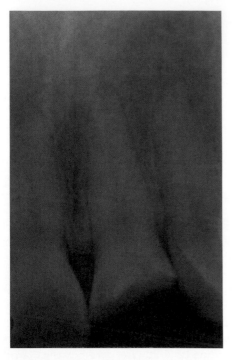

Figure 1.1   Pre-op radiograph of fractured tooth #9.

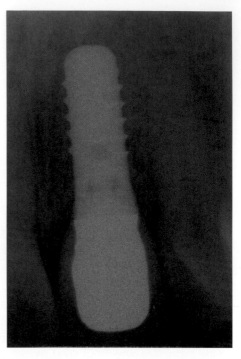

Figure 1.3   Final radiograph of immediate implant replacing tooth #9.

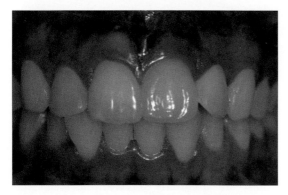

Figure 1.2   Final restoration of immediate implant replacing tooth #9.

necessary to incorporate immediate implant placement into their modality of patient care. Certainly not exhaustive in terms of literature, this text references the classic and contemporary scientific articles that provide the foundation for the art and science of this important

clinical topic. For some, these pages will begin their journey into a fascinating area of implant dentistry, while for others these written words will serve to reinforce and challenge their clinical expertise.

References

Barzilay, I. (1993). "Immediate implants: Their current status." *Int J Prosthodont* 6(2): 169–175.

Chen, S. T., J. Beagle, et al. (2009). "Consensus statements and recommended clinical procedures regarding surgical techniques." *Int J Oral Maxillofac Implants* 24 Suppl: 272–278.

Chen, S. T., T. G. Wilson, Jr., et al. (2004). "Immediate or early placement of implants following tooth extraction: Review of biologic basis, clinical procedures, and outcomes." *Int J Oral Maxillofac Implants* 19 Suppl: 12–25.

Denissen, H. W., W. Kalk, et al. (1993). "Anatomic consideration for preventive implantation." *Int J Oral Maxillofac Implants* 8(2): 191–196.

Gelb, D. A. (1993). "Immediate implant surgery: Three-year retrospective evaluation of 50 consecutive cases." *Int J Oral Maxillofac Implants* 8(4): 388–399.

Lazzara, R. J. (1989). "Immediate implant placement into extraction sites: Surgical and restorative advantages." *Int J Periodontics Restorative Dent* 9(5): 332–343.

Mayfield, L., ed. (1999). *Immediate, Delayed, and Late Submerged and Transmucosal Implants.* Berlin: Quintessence.

Missika, P., M. Abbou, et al. (1997). "Osseous regeneration in immediate postextraction implant placement: A literature review and clinical evaluation." *Pract Periodontics Aesthet Dent* 9(2): 165–175; quiz 176.

Parel, S. M., and R. G. Triplett (1990). "Immediate fixture placement: A treatment planning alternative." *Int J Oral Maxillofac Implants* 5(4): 337–345.

Schulte, W., and G. Heimke (1976). "[The Tübinger immediate implant]." *Quintessenz* 27(6): 17–23.

Schultz, A. J. (1993). "Guided tissue regeneration (GTR) of nonsubmerged implants in immediate extraction sites." *Pract Periodontics Aesthet Dent* 5(2): 59–65; quiz 66.

Schwartz-Arad, D., and G. Chaushu (1997). "Placement of implants into fresh extraction sites: 4 to 7 years retrospective evaluation of 95 immediate implants." *J Periodontol* 68(11): 1110–1116.

Shanaman, R. H. (1992). "The use of guided tissue regeneration to facilitate ideal prosthetic placement of implants." *Int J Periodontics Restorative Dent* 12(4): 256–265.

Watzek, G., R. Haider, et al. (1995). "Immediate and delayed implantation for complete restoration of the jaw following extraction of all residual teeth: A retrospective study comparing different types of serial immediate implantation." *Int J Oral Maxillofac Implants* 10(5): 561–567.

Werbitt, M. J., and P. V. Goldberg (1992). "The immediate implant: Bone preservation and bone regeneration." *Int J Periodontics Restorative Dent* 12(3): 206–217.

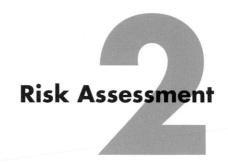

Risk Assessment

Implant dentistry requires the execution of a thorough treatment plan to obtain an ideal result for the patient. Although a proposed implant site may initially appear straight-forward, the clinician should be aware that there is nothing "simple" about outcomes with dental implants. This is certainly true regarding treatment plans in the esthetic zone and especially valid with regards to immediate implant placement. The clinician's primary goal should be to provide the patient with the highest level of outcome possible with the least degree of risk or complications (Dawson, Chen, et al. 2009). With this as the endpoint, several primary factors should be evaluated. These include the judgment and experience of the dentist, the local and systemic factors of the patient, and the bio-mechanics of the chosen implant system and grafting materials (Figure 2.1). Together, comprehensive evaluation of these factors will empower the dental team toward obtaining an ideal outcome.

SURGEON

It is clear that implant dentistry is not "easy." Not only is the dental team responsible for achieving a perfect esthetic, functional, and phonetic outcome, but it is also often responsible for the reconstruction of the alveolar bone and peri-implant soft tissues. This is often the case with immediate placement procedures (Figures 2.2–2.5).

As a mechanism to assist dental teams with their understanding of treatment planning, the Swiss Society of Oral Implantology (SSOI) and the International Team for Implantology (ITI) have adapted the SAC classification for surgical and prosthetic applications for implant dentistry with S=Straightforward, A=Advanced, and C=Complex (Dawson, Chen, et al. 2009) (Tables 2.1–2.4). From discussions in this classification system, immediate placement is to be considered "complex" and treatment should be limited to those surgeons with significant experience in implant procedures,

Surgical Essentials of Immediate Implant Dentistry, First Edition. Jay R. Beagle.
© 2013 John Wiley & Sons, Inc. Published 2013 by John Wiley & Sons, Inc.

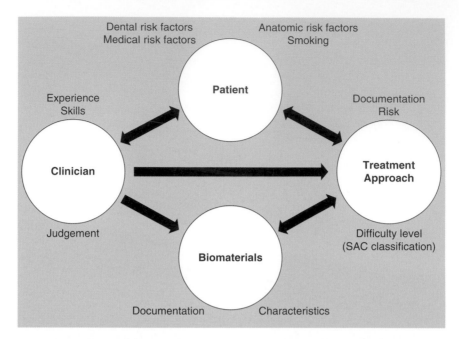

Figure 2.1 Decision tree for implant dentistry. From *ITI Treatment Guide*, vol. 3. Courtesy of Quintessence Publishing.

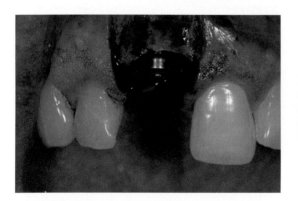

Figure 2.2 Immediate implant having thin buccal plate.

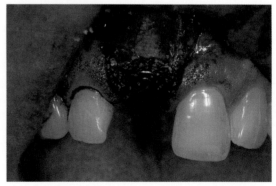

Figure 2.4 Buccal view of defect filled with autogenous bone.

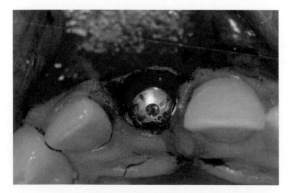

Figure 2.3 Large horizontal defect associated with an immediate implant following placement.

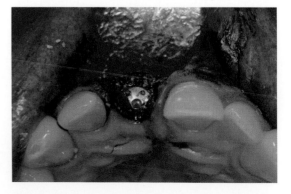

Figure 2.5 Occlusal view of defect filled with autogenous bone.

Table 2.1 Surgical SAC classification table.

	Straightforward	Advanced	Complex
Sufficient Bone Volume	Edentulous mandible Single posterior tooth Free-end posterior	Single tooth maxilla Large gap maxilla Tissue grafting Esthetics	Full arch maxilla/ mandible
Bone Deficiencies		Fenestration/dehiscence Sinus elevation Lateral augmentation	Extended defects Lateral/vertical augmentation Osseodistraction Extraoral harvesting

Table 2.2 SAC straightforward surgical recommendations.

Surgery—Straightforward

Simple surgical intervention
No anatomical risk
No surgical risk
Low complications
Sufficient bone quantity
Sufficient vertical/horizontal dimensions

Table 2.3 SAC advanced surgical recommendations.

Surgery—Advanced

Challenging surgical intervention
Anatomical risk
Little surgical risk
Possible complications
Single tooth esthetic gap in maxilla
Osteotome sinus lift
Simultaneous membrane technique

Table 2.4 SAC complex surgical recommendations.

Surgery—Complex

Complicated surgical intervention
Anatomical risk
High surgical demands
Expected complications
Edentulous maxilla
Bilateral sinus grafting
Vertical augmentation
Graft harvesting
Complex soft tissue grafting
High esthetic demands
Immediate implant placement/loading

hard and soft tissue grafting, extractions, and handling early and late complications. This increased level of surgical knowledge and expertise will complement the actual physical assessment of the patient from a medical, dental, and psychological viewpoint. The complex nature of immediate placement represents a challenge to the most experienced clinicians, requiring significant skills, competence, and knowledge should a complication arise.

PATIENT

Assessing the individual risk profile of a patient is critical when developing a dental treatment plan for both conventional and implant dentistry. There are many situations that arise that will direct a seemingly straightforward implant treatment plan into a non-implant approach for a patient. This stems from the fact that the assessment of a patient for implant treatment is multi-factorial, involving two basic concerns: systemic risk and local risk (Dawson, Chen, et al. 2009). Systemic risk includes the medical and physiological well-being of a patient, while local risk involves dental and anatomic-related issues. Appropriate evaluation and assessment of these risk factors or indicators will help the clinician avoid unnecessary post-treatment complications and assist in providing the patient with the desired outcome.

SYSTEMIC RISK

Much has been written in the literature regarding the medical health of a patient who is being evaluated for implant surgery. It is important to recognize those diseases or conditions that negatively impact the wound healing, bone remodeling, and long-term maintenance of osseointegrated implants with which a patient presents. Systemic contraindications for dental implant surgery have been divided into two main groups: very high-risk (group 1) and significant risk (group 2) (Buser, von Arx, et al. 2000). Very high-risk patients are those who present with serious systemic diseases (rheumatoid arthritis, osteomalecia, osteogenesis imperfecta); immunocompromised patients (HIV, immunosuppressed medications); use of intravenous bisphosphonates; drug and alcohol abusers; and non-compliant patients (including psychological and mental disorders) (Table 2.5). Significant risk patients include those who have irradiated bone (radiotherapy); severe diabetes;

Table 2.5 High-risk table.

Very High Risk
Rheumatoid arthritis
Osteomalecia
Osteogenesis imperfecta
HIV
Immunosuppressed medications
IV bisphosphonates
Drug and alcohol abuse
Psychological disorders
Mental disorders

bleeding disorders (hemorrhagic diathesis, drug-induced anticoagulation); and heavy smoking habit (Table 2.6). It is important that risks for implant failure and risks for medical complications should be differentiated and evaluated. In some instances, medical conditions and their treatments may pose an increased

Table 2.6 Significant risk table.

Significant Risk
Radiation therapy
Severe diabetes
Hemorrhagic diathesis
Drug-induced anticoagulation
Heavy smoking habit

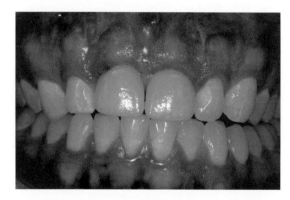

Figure 2.6 Buccal view illustrating a thick gingival phenotype.

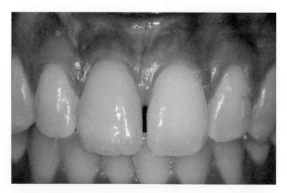

Figure 2.7 Buccal view illustrating a thin gingival phenotype.

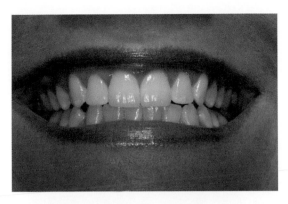

Figure 2.8 Buccal view of excellent periodontal health.

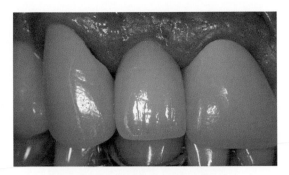

Figure 2.10 Final restoration of immediate implant replacing tooth #7.

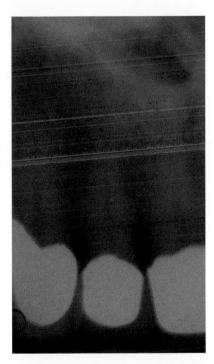

Figure 2.9 Presence of adjacent restorations prior to implant placement for tooth #7.

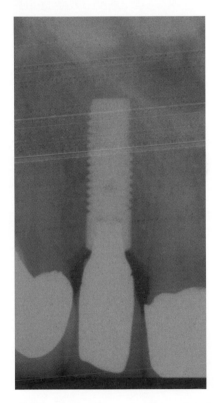

Figure 2.11 Final radiograph of immediate implant replacing tooth #7.

risk for implant failure, whereas the risk for the patient may be minimal.

When planning for the immediate placement of dental implants, local risk factors involving dental and anatomic issues require assessment. Regardless of the tooth site, the patients should be assessed for growth considerations (in adolescents/young adults), gingival phenotype (Figures 2.6 and 2.7), periodontal health (Figure 2.8), restorative/endodontic status of neighboring teeth (Figures 2.9–2.14), bone level

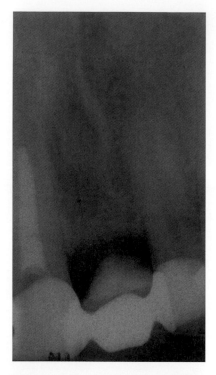

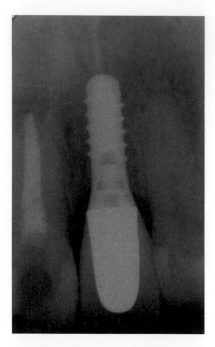

Figure 2.14   Final radiograph of tooth #10.

Figure 2.12   Healthy endodontic status of adjacent teeth prior to implant placement of tooth #10.

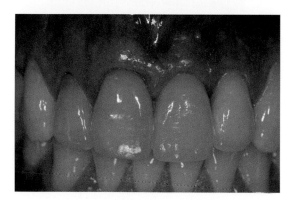

Figure 2.13   Final restoration of tooth #10.

of adjacent teeth (Figures 2.15–2.17), relationship of the socket/root apex to the sinus floor and inferior alveolar nerve (Figure 2.18), the presence of a malocclusion benefiting from orthodontic therapy (Figure 2.19), bone volume (Figure 2.20), width of the site to be restored,

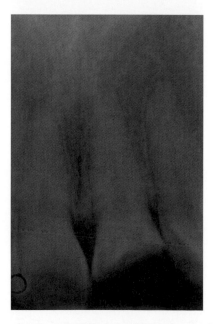

Figure 2.15   Favorable crestal bone levels of adjacent teeth prior to immediate implant placement for tooth #9.

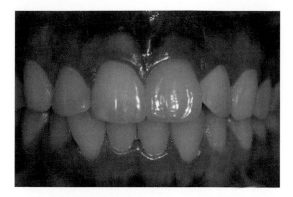

Figure 2.16 Final restoration of immediate implant replacing tooth #9.

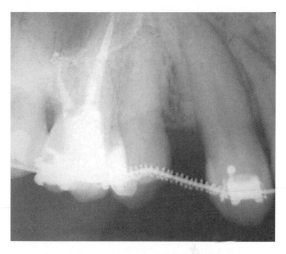

Figure 2.19 Root proximity of adjacent teeth requiring orthodontic treatment prior to implant treatment.

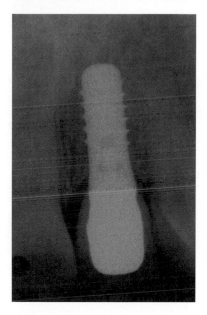

Figure 2.17 Final radiograph of immediate implant replacing tooth #9.

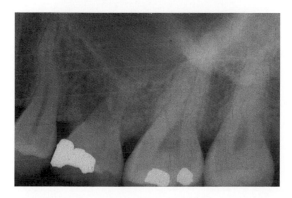

Figure 2.18 Proximity of sinus floor to deciduous tooth K.

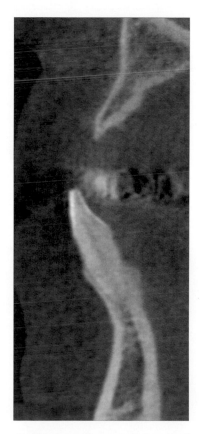

Figure 2.20 Cone beam CT image illustrating reduced bone volume.

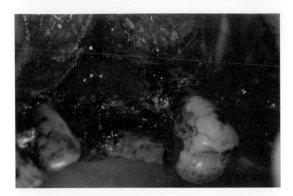

Figure 2.21   Presence of an osseous infection requiring staged bone grafting prior to implant placement.

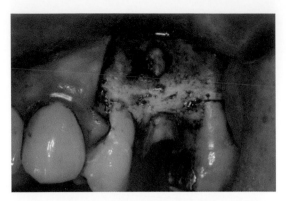

Figure 2.24   Buccal view of a fenestration defect at the apex of tooth #13.

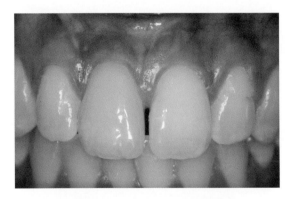

Figure 2.22   Buccal view of a thin gingival phenotype with a tapered crown morphology.

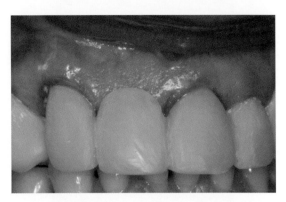

Figure 2.25   Provisional fixed partial denture utilized while the implant replacing tooth #8 osseointegrates.

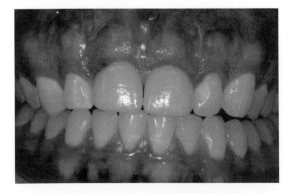

Figure 2.23   Buccal view of a thick gingival phenotype with a square crown morphology.

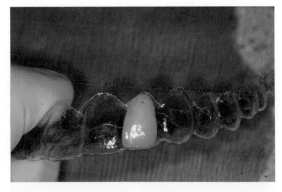

Figure 2.26   Fabrication of an Essix appliance replacing tooth #10.

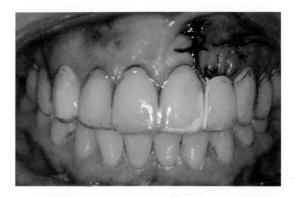

Figure 2.27 Buccal view of an Essix appliance replacing tooth #10.

and the presence of a significant osseous infection (Figure 2.21) (Dawson, Chen, et al. 2009).

Immediate placement involving the esthetic zone should also evaluate the patient's esthetic expectations, smile/lip line, crown shape, gingival architecture (Figures 2.22 and 2.23), thickness of the facial boney plate, presence of a fenestration or dehiscence-type defect (Figure 2.24), and the method of provisionaliza tion during the phase of osseointegration (Figures 2.25–2.27) (Dawson, Chen, et al. 2009).

BIOMATERIALS

The placement of immediate dental implants is unquestionably a challenge to the surgeon regardless of the implant site. The architecture of the socket to be treated can have many variables, such as width/length relationship, the presence of dehiscences/fenestrations, interocclusal height restrictions, the relationship to adjacent teeth, and available bone quality/quantity. For these reasons, it is important that the clinician select the appropriate biomaterials that have been well documented in experimental and clinical studies to reduce the risk for complications and/or failure, and to assist in ensuring an excellent outcome. Biomaterials that are often needed with immediate placement protocols include the implant, barrier

membranes, and bone grafts and/or fillers (Gelb 1993; Becker, Dahlin, et al. 1994; Zitzmann, Scharer, et al. 1999; Hammerle and Lang 2001; Schropp, Wenzel, et al. 2003).

IMPLANT DESIGN

One of the essential requirements for success with immediate implant placement is the ability to initially achieve primary stability. Equally important, however, is the maintenance of bone height/width following osseointegration and restoration. It is paramount, therefore, to select an implant design to benefit both goals (Figure 2.28).

To date, the following features remain important (Chen, Wilson, et al. 2004):

Implant Shape:
- Threaded design
- Cylindrical or hybrid taper shape
- Various length/width combinations
- Thread geometry/pitch to provide primary stability
- Bone-level platform for anterior placement
- Tissue-level platform for posterior placement

Abutment/Implant Connection:
- Internal connection
- Vertical or horizontal platform shift
- Long connection for stability

Prosthetic Components:
- Available CAD/CAM components
- Titanium, gold cast-to, or zirconium

Implant Surface:
- Micro-roughened texture
- Bioactive

One of the key factors in selecting an implant and restorative components is the scientific commitment, stability, and longevity of the manufacturer. It is important to utilize a product with excellent experimental and clinical research, innovative concepts, and customer service. It is not unusual today to encounter

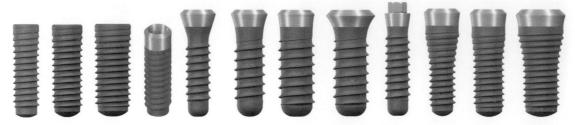

Figure 2.28 Current Straumann implants available for 2012. Images courtesy of Straumann USA, LLC, its parents, affiliates or subsidiaries. © Straumann USA LLC, all rights reserved.

patients requiring new abutments/crowns on antiquated implant styles, only to find that the needed components are no longer available.

BARRIER MEMBRANES

Barrier membranes have long-term documentation in experimental animal trials, histologic studies, and human clinical trials supporting their value in bone regeneration. Initially utilized for guided tissue regeneration (GTR) for the regeneration of lost attachment in periodontal defects, barrier membranes take on the following roles with immediate implant placement (Figures 2.29–2.36):

1. Prevention of epithelial downgrowth into the vertical/horizontal defect associated with the implant site
2. Protection of osseous grafts
3. Protection of the labial plate from resorption following implant placement

Originally, barrier membranes consisted of non-resorbable ePTFE requiring a second surgery for retrieval. Often, these membranes became secondarily infected if prematurely exposed and resulted in diminished regenerative outcomes. Today, the following barrier membrane characteristics are valuable with immediate implant placement procedures:

- Bioresorbability
- Lack of foreign body reaction
- +3-month duration before resorbing

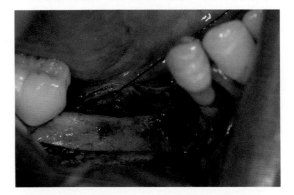

Figure 2.29 Buccal view of socket defect and edentulous ridge defect.

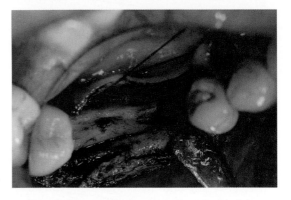

Figure 2.30 Occlusal view of socket defect and edentulous ridge defect.

- hydrophilic
- stiffness
- adaptability
- no need for recovery
- minimal susceptibility for infection

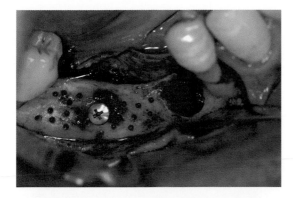

Figure 2.31 Buccal view of decorticated ridge and fixation screw.

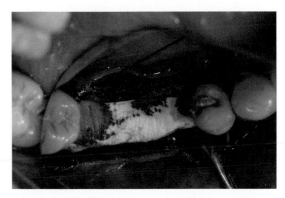

Figure 2.34 Occlusal view of edentulous ridge treated with an allograft and resorbable membrane.

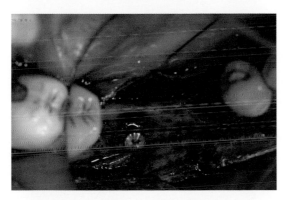

Figure 2.32 Occlusal view of decorticated ridge and fixation screw.

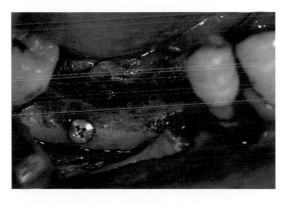

Figure 2.35 Buccal view illustrating 6-month post-operative result of guided bone regeneration.

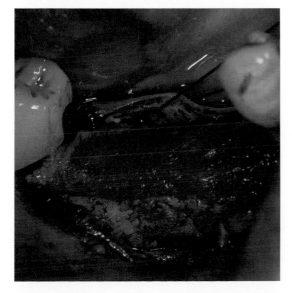

Figure 2.33 Buccal view of edentulous ridge treated with an allograft and resorbable membrane.

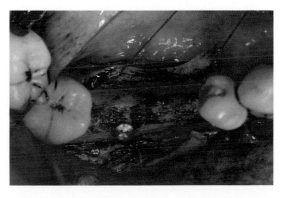

Figure 2.36 Occlusal view illustrating 6-month post-operative result of guided bone regeneration.

BONE GRAFTS (FILLERS)

Quite often with immediate implant placement, a vertical or horizontal gap occurs between the socket wall and implant surface (Figures 2.37 and 2.38). This is particularly desired along the labial plate to avoid compression necrosis of the boney wall. Experimental and clinical studies have shown that a horizontal gap measuring less than 2 mm will regenerate as long as a blood clot forms and is not disrupted. Bone grafts have proven helpful with more extensive horizontal and vertical gaps to expedite osseo-integration and provide shorter intervals for healing, as well as to provide support to barrier membranes and prevent their collapse into the defect. Autogenous coagulum and chips were originally recommended for this function; however, new products have been developed as alternatives to autogenous grafts to simplify

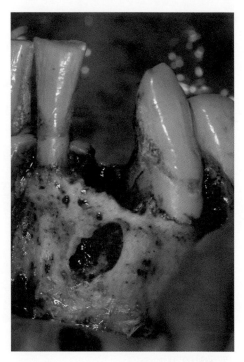

Figure 2.39 Buccal view of fenestration defect prior to the placement of an immediate implant for tooth #23.

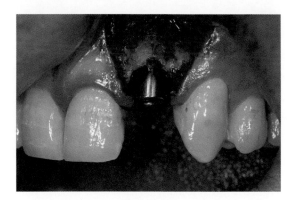

Figure 2.37 Buccal view of crestal defect following immediate implant placement.

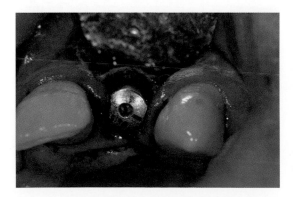

Figure 2.38 Occlusal view of crestal defect following immediate implant placement.

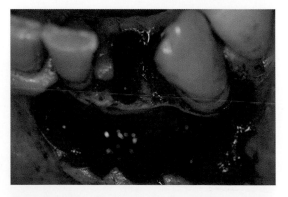

Figure 2.40 Occlusal view of fenestration defect prior to the placement of an immediate implant for tooth #23.

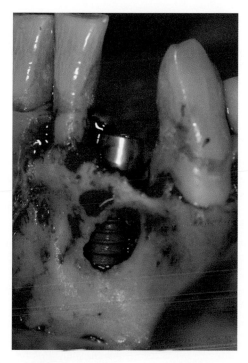

Figure 2.41 Buccal view of immediate implant placement for tooth #23,

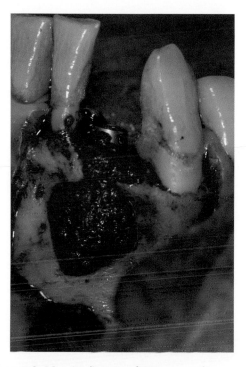

Figure 2.43 Application of autogenous bone graft into fenestration defect and crestal defect.

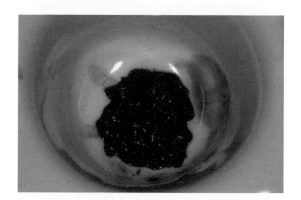

Figure 2.42 Autogenous bone graft obtained during osteotomy preparation for immediate implant placement.

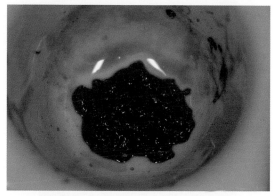

Figure 2.44 Xenograft hydrated with blood.

surgical procedures for the clinician and reduce patient morbidity and risk (Figures 2.39–2.46). Autogenous grafts are still considered the standard for small implant defects, but when utilized, non-autogenous grafts should have the following characteristics:

- Minimal foreign body reaction
- Osteoconductivity
- Low substitution rate
- Favorable particulate size
- Ease of handling
- Cost-effectiveness

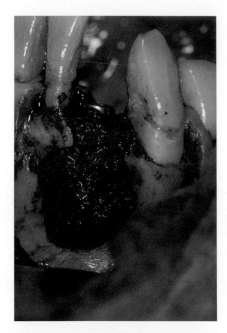

Figure 2.45 Application of xenograft as a veneer over the autogenous bone graft.

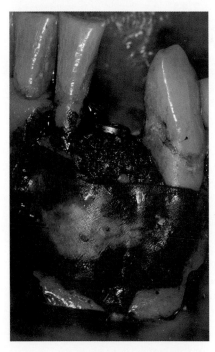

Figure 2.46 Placement of a resorbable membrane over the bone graft materials.

It is important to keep the osseous grafting materials hydrated prior to use with blood, sterile water, or growth factor, per the manufacturer's recommendations, which have been proven experimentally, histologically, and/or in clinical studies.

References

Becker, W., C. Dahlin, et al. (1994). "The use of e-PTFE barrier membranes for bone promotion around titanium implants placed into extraction sockets: A prospective multicenter study." *Int J Oral Maxillofac Implants* 9(1): 31–40.

Buser, D., T. von Arx, et al. (2000). "Basic surgical principles with ITI implants." *Clin Oral Implants Res* 11 Suppl 1: 59–68.

Chen, S. T., T. G. Wilson, Jr., et al. (2004). "Immediate or early placement of implants following tooth extraction: Review of biologic basis, clinical procedures, and outcomes." *Int J Oral Maxillofac Implants* 19 Suppl: 12–25.

Dawson, A., S. Chen, et al. (2009). *The SAC Classification in Implant Dentistry*. Berlin: Quintessence.

Gelb, D. A. (1993). "Immediate implant surgery: Three-year retrospective evaluation of 50 consecutive cases." *Int J Oral Maxillofac Implants* 8(4): 388–399.

Hammerle, C. H., and N. P. Lang (2001). "Single stage surgery combining transmucosal implant placement with guided bone regeneration and bioresorbable materials." *Clin Oral Implants Res* 12(1): 9–18.

Schropp, L., A. Wenzel, et al. (2003). "Bone healing and soft tissue contour changes following single-tooth extraction: A clinical and radiographic 12-month prospective study." *Int J Periodontics Restorative Dent* 23(4): 313–323.

Zitzmann, N. U., P. Scharer, et al. (1999). "Factors influencing the success of GBR: Smoking, timing of implant placement, implant location, bone quality and provisional restoration." *J Clin Periodontol* 26(10): 673–682.

Indications and Contraindications

The placement of immediate dental implants can provide a similar success/survival outcome as that of early and delayed placement protocols, as long as attention is given to several critical guidelines (Chen, Wilson, et al. 2004; Wagenberg and Froum 2006; Chen, Beagle, et al. 2009). These guidelines can be considered as indications and contraindications for immediate placement and are represented by a number of clinical and anatomic challenges with which the patient may present.

As previously discussed in the chapter concerning risk assessment, a number of local factors involving dental and anatomic issues must be assessed before surgical placement of immediate dental implants (Chen and Buser 2009). Failure of the dentist to thoroughly address these localized issues may result in an outcome that is deemed unsatisfactory with regards to esthetics or function and may prevent the implant from achieving osseointegration (Figure 3.1). Quite often, both the dentist and the patient become too focused on replacing a failing tooth

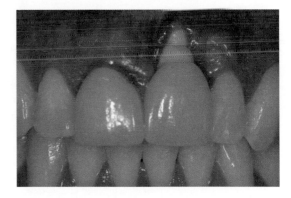

Figure 3.1 Unsatisfactory esthetics with tooth #9 implant.

with an immediate implant to accelerate the treatment process, only to arrive at the endpoint with an unforeseen complication that could have been avoided with a better understanding of the treatment complexities (Chen and Buser 2009). This chapter will focus on the local risk factors commonly encountered with the surgical placement of immediate dental implants.

Surgical Essentials of Immediate Implant Dentistry, First Edition. Jay R. Beagle.
© 2013 John Wiley & Sons, Inc. Published 2013 by John Wiley & Sons, Inc.

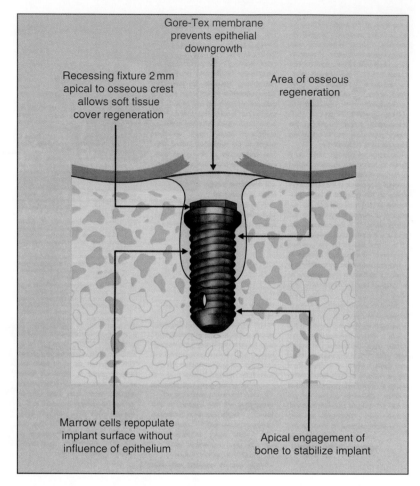

Figure 3.2   Original diagram of immediate placement protocol. From Lazzara 1989. Courtesy of Quintessence Publishing.

PRIMARY STABILITY

Along with proper restoratively driven positioning, the ability to achieve primary mechanical stability with an immediately placed dental implant is paramount (Figure 3.2) (Lazzara 1989). Often this requires the implant to engage bone along the lateral walls of the socket without changing the original socket depth, or by engaging bone apical to the original socket dimensions. In either of these situations, only one to three threads of the implant need to be in contact with the osteot-

omy site. An implant that can be moved laterally with finger pressure following placement will have a poor chance of achieving osseointegration and should be aborted. Care should be exercised to follow the manufacturer's preparation guidelines, as an undersized osteotomy may result in compression necrosis of the bone, thus causing implant failure to occur (Figures 3.3–3.5). This is especially true with the use of tapered designed implants when the primary stability is developed at the crest, rather than apically or laterally. Another frequent mishap in an effort to achieve primary stability is choosing an implant with a

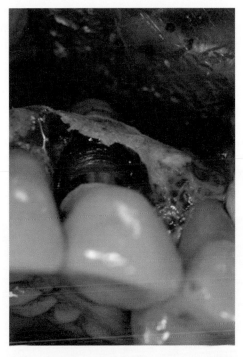

Figure 3.3 Occlusal view of bone loss caused by compression necrosis.

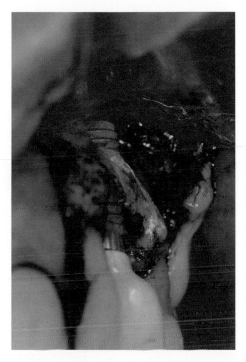

Figure 3.5 Lateral view of bone loss caused by compression necrosis.

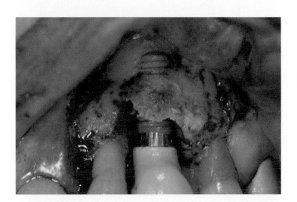

Figure 3.4 Buccal view of bone loss caused by compression necrosis.

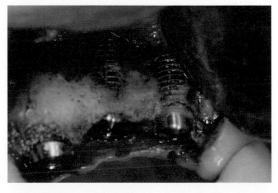

Figure 3.6 Loss of buccal plate caused by selecting improper implant diameter.

restorative platform too large for the planned restoration, only because the larger implant diameter is able to achieve stability. Not only is this a concern for esthetics, but a larger implant diameter may not provide sufficient space between the implant surface and the buccal plate

(horizontal defect dimension, or HDD) to allow a blood clot to form or bone graft to be placed, and will therefore contribute to compression along the buccal plate of bone (Figure 3.6) (Buser, Martin, et al. 2004; Araujo, Wennstrom, et al. 2006).

INFERIOR ALVEOLAR NERVE

As with early and delayed placement, it is important to precisely locate the position of the inferior alveolar nerve, or the mental foramen, radiographically when placing an immediate implant in the posterior mandible. Many guidelines have been established that alert the clinician to stay at least 2 mm superior to the inferior alveolar nerve during the osteotomy and placement of the implant (Buser, von Arx, et al. 2000). Mandibular second premolar sites frequently have their apex near the mental foramen and also have a wide socket morphology requiring a 4.8 mm implant diameter for stability (Figure 3.7). In some instances, it may be best to proceed with an early placement protocol, rather than immediate, for these situations where there is risk in injury to the nerve in an attempt to achieve primary stability.

The variability of root morphology for mandibular first and second molars makes immediate implant placement in these sites unpredictable. One should avoid the temptation to place the implant into the mesial or distal root socket to achieve stability, only to have an implant that results in poor positioning from a restorative perspective. It is often best to proceed with a 12-week healing period following the extraction of a mandibular molar before implant placement is performed (Chen, Wilson, et al. 2004). If an immediate molar implant can be placed, grafting the HDD with an osseous graft and use of a bioresorbable membrane will be required (Fugazzotto 2008a, 2008b), and a healing time to achieve osseointegration may exceed 16 weeks (Figures 3.8 and 3.9).

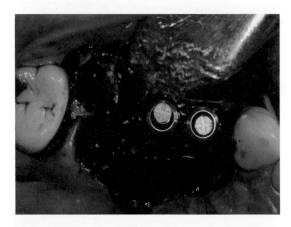

Figure 3.8 Occlusal view of tooth #3 following extraction and osteotomy preparation.

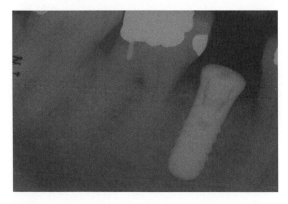

Figure 3.7 Radiograph of tooth #29 treated with immediate placement using a 4.8 mm diameter implant.

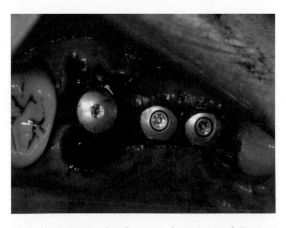

Figure 3.9 Occlusal view of tooth #3 following immediate placement.

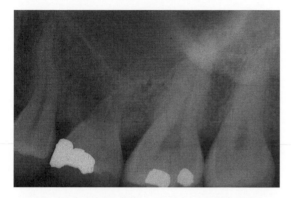

Figure 3.10 Radiograph of deciduous tooth K and the proximity to the maxillary sinus floor.

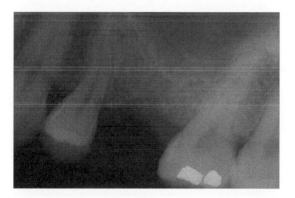

Figure 3.11 Radiograph of 12 weeks of healing following the extraction of tooth K.

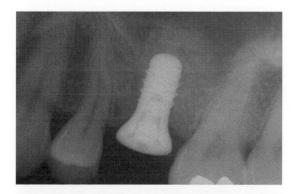

Figure 3.12 Radiograph of implant placed into the deciduous tooth K site in conjunction with a simultaneous osteotomy sinus lift and bone graft.

MAXILLARY SINUS

The maxillary sinus position may pose concerns when placing an immediate implant into the second premolar or first and second molar sites (Fugazzotto and De 2002). At times the second premolar site is circumferentially wide and primary stability cannot be achieved using a 4.8 mm diameter implant to engage the lateral walls of the socket. In these instances, an early placement protocol is desired to reduce the socket dimensions and provide stability and predictability (Figures 3.10–3.12). Similar to mandibular molar sites, it is desirable not to place a maxillary implant into the mesial-buccal, distal-buccal, or palatal root areas to gain primary stability, only to have an implant positioned poorly from a restorative perspective. Certainly, if adequate bone height is available in maxillary molar sites without penetration into the sinus, an immediate implant can be inserted, but these circumstances do not occur frequently.

SITES REQUIRING GUIDED BONE REGENERATION

Sites affected by trauma or infection may demonstrate significant loss in the buccal or lingual boney plates, thus exposing a significant amount of implant surface upon immediate placement. Although primary stability can be achieved, it is best to initiate guided bone regeneration (GBR) to reconstruct the alveolar ridge to improve success and optimize esthetics, especially in the anterior region (Figures 3.13 and 3.14) (Buser, Dula, et al. 1993; Buser, Bornstein, et al. 2008; Buser, Chen, et al. 2008). The predictability of GBR is well supported in the literature using autogenous bone grafts, bone morphogenic protein (BMP), or bone allografts in conjunction with membranes or titanium mesh for this indication (Buser, Dahlin, et al. 1994).

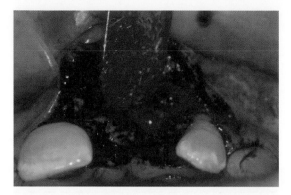

Figure 3.13 Occlusal view of #9 site requiring GBR.

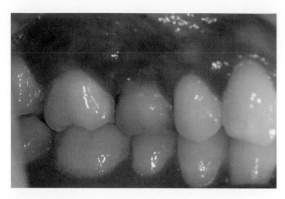

Figure 3.15 Buccal view of retained deciduous tooth A.

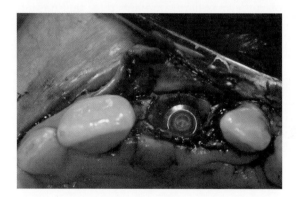

Figure 3.14 Occlusal view of #9 site following GBR.

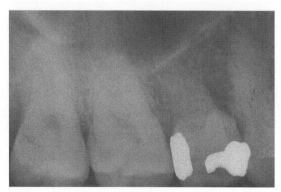

Figure 3.16 Radiograph of retained deciduous tooth A.

RETAINED DECIDUOUS TEETH

Retained deciduous teeth with a congenitally missing permanent tooth are often good candidates for an immediately placed implant (de Oliveira, Macedo, et al. 2009; Borzabadi-Farahani 2011). Frequently seen clinically is the absence of a maxillary or mandibular second premolar, with the retained deciduous molar in place (Figures 3.15–3.18). When detected early, these sites can be developed orthodontically to achieve the ideal mesial-distal dimension of the congenitally absent tooth prior to extraction. Following the cessation of alveolar jaw growth, the deciduous tooth can be removed and the implant inserted, assuming the anatomical

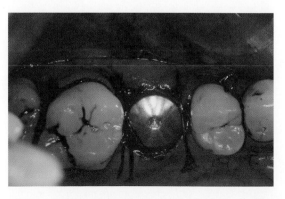

Figure 3.17 Occlusal view of immediate implant replacing deciduous tooth A.

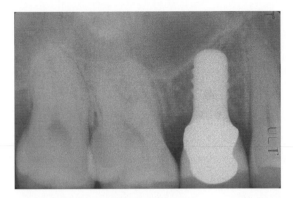

Figure 3.18   Final radiograph of immediate implant replacing deciduous tooth A.

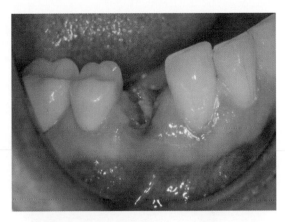

Figure 3.19   Buccal view of tooth #28 with non-restorable caries.

structures (alveolar nerve/sinus) are not at risk. Generally, adequate bone is available for primary implant stability to be achieved, even if the roots of the deciduous tooth are not fully resorbed. Minimal bone grafting and use of a resorbable membrane may be desired if an osseous defect is present in the residual root sockets, adjacent to the implant surface.

NON-RESTORABLE CARIOUS TEETH

Until recently, a periodontal crown-lengthening procedure or orthodontic extrusion was the primary treatment option available for teeth having significant subgingival caries (Rosenberg, Garber, et al. 1980; Sabri 1989). While both options are predictable, they result in esthetic concerns, especially in the maxillary anterior region. Periodontal crown-lengthening procedures often create a gingival asymmetry with an adjacent or contra-lateral tooth, as well as sacrifice alveolar crestal bone. Orthodontic extrusion can result in the need for gingival or osseous recontouring and also result in a tooth with a more constricted cervical contour. Extracting a tooth with severe subgingival caries offers the surgeon the opportunity to preserve the crestal bone and associated gingival

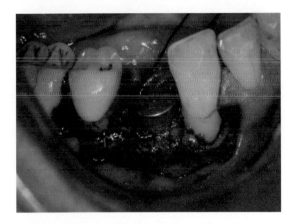

Figure 3.20   Buccal view of immediate placement for tooth #28.

tissues when an immediate implant is placed (Figures 3.19 and 3.20). Generally, achieving primary stability in these sites is not difficult, as the surrounding alveolus is intact. The immediate placement technique for this application may also be more cost-effective for the patient, considering the treatment needed to save the tooth involves periodontics, restorative dentistry, endodontics, and possibly orthodontics. As with previous indications, care must be exercised relative to risks of injury to vital anatomic structures, as well as having a restoratively driven placement.

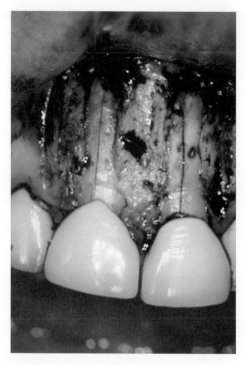

Figure 3.21 Buccal view of vertical root fractures.

VERTICAL/HORIZONTAL ROOT FRACTURES

Vertical and horizontal root fractures are most commonly seen with endodontically treated teeth (Fuss, Lustig, et al. 1999) and are considered non-treatable, with an exception of molars, which may often be treated with a root resection procedure. Teeth with root fractures are good candidates for an immediate placement protocol, assuming primary stability and ideal positioning can be achieved (Figure 3.21) (Becker, Becker, et al. 2000). The clinician should be aware that teeth that have been fractured for many weeks may be associated with an osseous defect appearing as a narrow or wide dehiscence. Following implant placement, if a dehiscence defect is present, it can be corrected with an osseous graft and resorbable membrane prior to flap closure (Buser, Wittneben, et al. 2011).

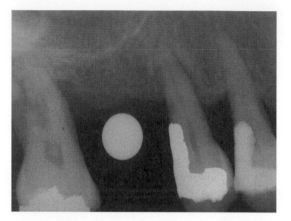

Figure 3.22 Radiograph of teeth with reduced periodontal support.

PERIODONTALLY INVOLVED TEETH

Unfortunately, clinicians are often faced with the issue of a patient with advanced periodontal disease or refractory disease that leads to tooth loss (Figure 3.22). Despite efforts to treat these sites, it may be inevitable that tooth loss will occur. In these situations, it is best to advise the patient to extract the affected tooth/teeth while enough alveolar bone is available for implant placement without risk of injury to the inferior alveolar nerve for mandibular posterior teeth (Wagenberg and Froum 2006; Hammerle, Araujo, et al. 2012). In these situations, it may be possible to place an immediate implant if the root morphology permits. Certainly the same concerns can be addressed for the maxillary posterior, while the ability to perform a sinus elevation procedure should allow for implant placement using a staged approach to treatment, if necessary.

LIP LINE

Many articles published in the dental literature report a higher incidence of marginal tissue recession associated with the placement

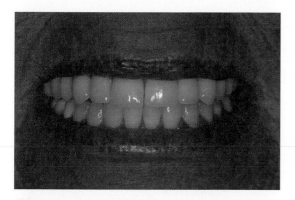

Figure 3.23 Illustration of a low smile line.

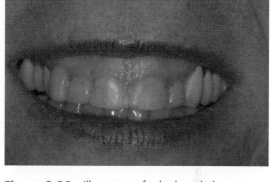

Figure 3.25 Illustration of a high smile line.

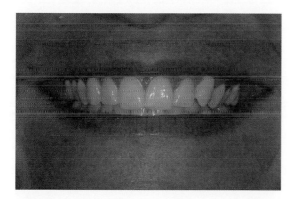

Figure 3.24 Illustration of a medium smile line.

of immediate dental implants (Cornelini, Cangini, et al. 2005; Barone, Rispoli, et al. 2006; Chen, Darby, et al. 2007; Kan, Rungcharassaeng, et al. 2007; Buser, Halbritter, et al. 2009; Chen, Beagle, et al. 2009). This may be related to a number of factors that are in control of the dental team involving hard and soft tissue augmentation, crown contour during provisionalization, accuracy of tissue reproduction during impressions, frenum attachments, and definitive crown contour (Buser, Martin, et al. 2004). Patients who present with a high lip line or broad esthetic zone need to be aware of the potential of a final restoration that may become asymmetric relative to the contra-lateral tooth as a result of these

issues (Belser, Martin, et al. 2007). Clearly immediate placement should be avoided in situations where potential marginal tissue recession cannot be controlled in a high smile line situation, assuming a staged approach could offer a more predictable outcome (Figures 3.23–3.25).

PATIENT EXPECTATIONS

Dentists frequently encounter the emotions displayed by a patient who has been told that he or she has a tooth requiring extraction. Upon hearing this news, most motivated patients wish to move through treatment as quickly as possible to avoid the esthetic or functional embarrassment of being partially edentulous, especially if it involves an anterior tooth.

It is important that the dental team understand the patient's desired esthetic expectations before initiating treatment in the event that local factors may require attention prior to implant placement to achieve the desired outcome (Garber and Belser 1995; Norton 2004). At the very minimum, the clinician should employ a risk factor chart (Table 3.1) when treatment planning immediate implants (Belser, Martin, et al. 2007).

Table 3.1   Table addressing esthetic risk.

Esthetic Risk Factors	Low Risk	Moderate Risk	High Risk
Medical Status	+ Immune		− Immune
Smoking Habit	None	<10 cigs/day	>10 cigs/day
Patient's Esthetic Expectations	Low	Medium	High
Lip Line	Low	Medium	High
Gingival Phenotype	Low, thick	Medium, thick	High, thin
Shape of Tooth Crowns	Rectangular		Triangular
Infection at Site	None	Chronic	Acute
Adjacent Tooth Bone Level	<5 mm	5.5–6.5 mm	>7 mm
Adjacent Tooth Restorative Status	Virgin	Minimal	Restored
Width of Edentulous Span	1 tooth >7 mm	1 tooth <7 mm	>2 teeth
Alveolar Crest Anatomy	No deficiency	Horiz. defect	Vert. defect
Timing of Implant Placement	T 4	T 2 & T 3	T 1

From *ITI Treatment Guide*, vol. 1. Courtesy of Quintessence Publishing.

TISSUE PHENOTYPE

The band of keratinized/attached tissue for dental implants and teeth along the buccal is referred to in terms of the patient having a thick or thin phenotype. Martin et al. have further added a classification of a medium phenotype (Belser, Martin, et al. 2007). These tissue phenotypes have specific visual and situational characteristics that may influence the esthetic and long-term stability of the soft tissues adjacent to dental implant restorations.

The most favorable phenotype for a clinician to control is the thick tissue phenotype (Figure 3.26) (Kan, Rungcharassaeng, et al. 2003; Kois 2004). This occurs in approximately 80% of the population and is noted as being composed of a broad (>4 mm) band of attached mucosa. Not surprisingly, this phenotype is the most resistant to marginal tissue recession and is able to mask the metallic color of the implant and associated restorative components, especially when the implant is positioned in a shallow dimension. The clinician should be aware that the thick tissue phenotype might be more prone to heal with scar formation when vertical releasing incisions are required to gain access to the surgical site.

Thin tissue phenotypes are less frequently encountered but present significant challenges to

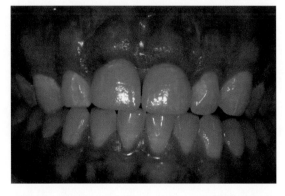

Figure 3.26 Illustration of a thick gingival phenotype.

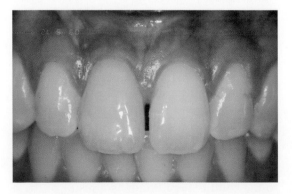

Figure 3.27 Illustration of a thin gingival phenotype.

the dental team (Figure 3.27). Thin phenotypes are comprised of a narrow zone of keratinized tissue and have been shown to have an increased risk of marginal tissue recession following restoration (Kan, Rungcharassaeng, et al. 2003; Kois 2004; Evans and Chen 2008). Sites exhibiting this phenotype benefit from hard and soft tissue augmentation at the time of implant placement, as well as positioning the implant slightly palatally. It is imperative that a fixed provisional restoration be constructed following osseointegration prior to obtaining a final impression for the definitive restoration. When properly handled, the esthetic outcome of a dental implant having a thin tissue phenotype can be outstanding, especially if the adjacent teeth are periodontally healthy and have unaltered crestal bone levels.

CRESTAL BONE LEVELS OF THE TREATMENT SITE AND ADJACENT TEETH

Pre-treatment soft and hard tissue relationships to adjacent teeth can affect the esthetic outcome

of immediate dental implants (Figures 3.28–3.30). A number of studies have shown the presence or absence of an interdental papilla is directly related to interproximal bone heights (Figures 3.31–3.35) (Choquet, Hermans, et al. 2001; Ryser, Block, et al. 2005). To improve those situations in which proximal bone loss has

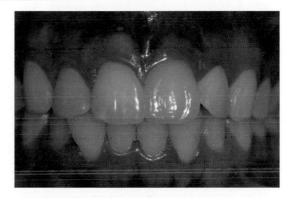

Figure 3.29 Final restoration of tooth #9 replacement with an immediate implant.

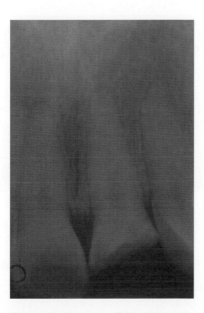

Figure 3.28 Radiograph of favorable crestal bone heights in replacing tooth #9 with an immediate implant.

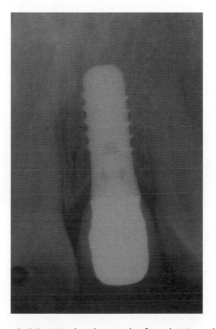

Figure 3.30 Final radiograph of tooth #9 replaced with an immediate implant.

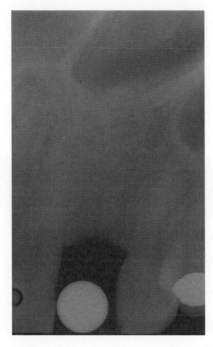

Figure 3.31 Radiograph of moderate-risk crestal bone levels for implant replacing tooth #10.

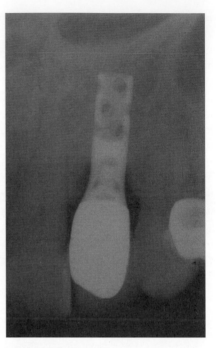

Figure 3.33 Final radiograph of implant replacing #10 with moderate-risk crestal bone levels.

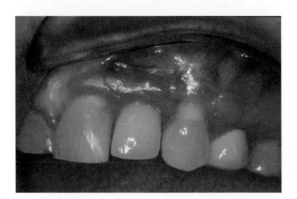

Figure 3.32 Final restoration of implant replacing tooth #10.

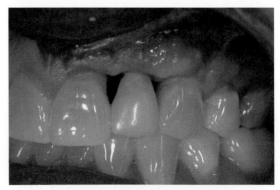

Figure 3.34 Final restoration of moderate implant replacing tooth #10 high-risk crestal bone levels.

occurred, orthodontic extrusion of the tooth to be extracted can be performed to enhance the esthetic outcome (Salama and Salama 1993).

This may require endodontic therapy to be performed on the treated tooth and obviously increases time and costs for the patient.

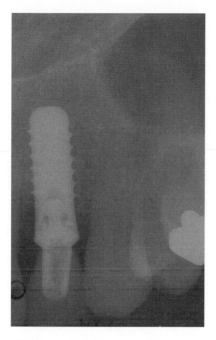

Figure 3.35 Final radiograph of implant replacing tooth #10 with high-risk crestal bone levels.

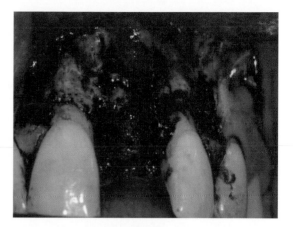

Figure 3.36 Buccal view of long dehiscence defect involving tooth #9.

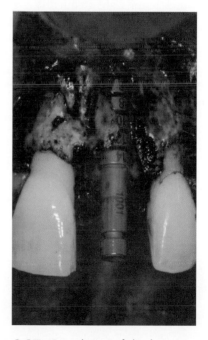

Figure 3.37 Buccal view of depth gauge in place during the treatment of tooth #9 with an immediate implant.

DEHISCENCE DEFECTS

Perhaps the greatest challenge with any dental implant procedure in the esthetic zone for a surgeon is to recreate a gingival profile that mimics that of a periodontally perfect contralateral tooth. One of the keys to success is managing the buccal bone crest, which will ultimately support the peri-implant soft tissues. As with soft tissue phenotypes, the buccal bone crest can be considered thick (>2mm) or thin (<1mm). Studies have shown that thin crestal bone will undergo significant resorption following tooth extraction and this may affect the position of the resultant soft tissue profile (Chen, Darby, et al. 2007; Kan, Rungcharassaeng, et al. 2007). It is often observed that these thin buccal bone crests are associated with a buccal bone dehiscence prior to tooth extraction (Rupprecht, Horning, et al. 2001) and frequently develop iatrogenically at the time of

tooth extraction, even with the most careful and experienced clinician.

The observation or occurrence of a buccal dehiscence (Figures 3.36 and 3.37) should not present an absolute contraindication to proceeding with an immediate placement procedure, but should require the clinician to reconstruct this defect using osseous grafts having a low substitution rate as well as bio-resorbable membranes at the time of implant placement (Buser, Wittneben, et al. 2011). A semi- or fully submerged flap closure will ensure the graft is well contained and can mature with minimal healing disturbances.

FENESTRATION DEFECTS

Unlike dehiscence defects, fenestration defects usually do not affect the esthetic outcome of immediate implant placement (Figure 3.38). Buccal fenestrations are frequently seen with sites having a recurrent periapical lesion or are encountered by inadvertently exceeding the preparation shape with a larger than necessary twist drill diameter (Becker, Ochsenbein, et al. 1997; Rupprecht, Horning, et al. 2001). Several studies have shown that a flapless approach to delayed or immediate implant placement can result in a high frequency of buccal plates developing fenestration defects (Dawson, Chen, et al. 2009). As a recommendation, a guided surgery technique employing cone beam CT (CBCT) radiography and a surgical guide should be utilized if a flapless approach

is planned with immediate placement (Brodala 2009; Hammerle, Stone, et al. 2009).

When encountered, a fenestration defect should be corrected with a combination of an osseous graft and resorbable membrane following implant placement and presents no contra-indications for immediate placement (Mayfield, Nobreus, et al. 1997).

LOCAL INFECTION AT THE IMPLANT SITE

Frequently, sites to be treated with immediately placed dental implants are affected with either acute or chronic localized infections. The literature has been controversial concerning this topic, and as a result, this subject will be discussed in a separate chapter.

References

Araujo, M. G., J. L. Wennstrom, et al. (2006). "Modeling of the buccal and lingual bone walls of fresh extraction sites following implant installation." *Clin Oral Implants Res* 17(6): 606–614.

Barone, A., L. Rispoli, et al. (2006). "Immediate restoration of single implants placed immediately after tooth extraction." *J Periodontol* 77(11): 1914–1920.

Becker, W., B. E. Becker, et al. (2000). "Retrospective case series analysis of the factors determining immediate implant placement." *Compend Contin Educ Dent* 21(10): 805–808, 810–811, 814 passim; quiz 820.

Becker, W., C. Ochsenbein, et al. (1997). "Alveolar bone anatomic profiles as measured from dry skulls: Clinical ramifications." *J Clin Periodontol* 24(10): 727–731.

Belser, U., W. Martin, et al. (2007). *Implant Therapy in the Esthetic Zone*. Berlin: Quintessence.

Borzabadi-Farahani, A. (2011). "Orthodontic considerations in restorative management of

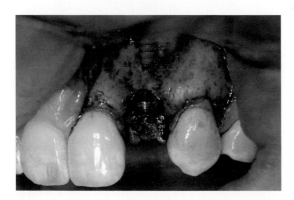

Figure 3.38 Buccal view of a fenestration defect following implant placement for tooth #10.

hypodontia patients with endosseous implants." *J Oral Implantol*. In press.

Brodala, N. (2009). "Flapless surgery and its effect on dental implant outcomes." *Int J Oral Maxillofac Implants* 24 Suppl: 118–125.

Buser, D., M. M. Bornstein, et al. (2008a). "Early implant placement with simultaneous guided bone regeneration following single-tooth extraction in the esthetic zone: A cross-sectional, retrospective study in 45 subjects with a 2- to 4-year follow-up." *J Periodontol* 79(9): 1773–1781.

Buser, D., S. T. Chen, et al. (2008b). "Early implant placement following single-tooth extraction in the esthetic zone: Biologic rationale and surgical procedures." *Int J Periodontics Restorative Dent* 28(5): 441–451.

Buser, D., C. Dahlin, et al., eds. (1994). *Guided Bone Regeneration in Implant Dentistry*. Berlin: Quintessence.

Buser, D., K. Dula, et al. (1993). "Localized ridge augmentation using guided bone regeneration. 1. Surgical procedure in the maxilla." *Int J Periodontics Restorative Dent* 13(1): 29–45.

Buser, D., S. Halbritter, et al. (2009). "Early implant placement with simultaneous guided bone regeneration following single-tooth extraction in the esthetic zone: 12-month results of a prospective study with 20 consecutive patients." *J Periodontol* 80(1): 152–162.

Buser, D., W. Martin, et al. (2004). "Optimizing esthetics for implant restorations in the anterior maxilla: Anatomic and surgical considerations." *Int J Oral Maxillofac Implants* 19 Suppl: 43–61.

Buser, D., T. von Arx, et al. (2000). "Basic surgical principles with ITI implants." *Clin Oral Implants Res* 11 Suppl 1: 59–68.

Buser, D., J. Wittneben, et al. (2011). "Stability of contour augmentation and esthetic outcomes of implant-supported single crowns in the esthetic zone: 3-year results of a prospective study with early implant placement postextraction." *J Periodontol* 82(3): 342–349.

Chen, S., and D. Buser (2009). *Implant Placement in Post-Extraction Sites*. Berlin: Quintessence.

Chen, S. T., J. Beagle, et al. (2009). "Consensus statements and recommended clinical procedures regarding surgical techniques." *Int J Oral Maxillofac Implants* 24 Suppl: 272–278.

Chen, S. T., I. B. Darby, et al. (2007). "A prospective clinical study of non-submerged immediate implants: Clinical outcomes and esthetic results." *Clin Oral Implants Res* 18(5): 552–562.

Chen, S. T., T. G. Wilson, Jr., et al. (2004). "Immediate or early placement of implants following tooth extraction: Review of biologic basis, clinical procedures, and outcomes." *Int J Oral Maxillofac Implants* 19 Suppl: 12–25.

Choquet, V., M. Hermans, et al. (2001). "Clinical and radiographic evaluation of the papilla level adjacent to single-tooth dental implants: A retrospective study in the maxillary anterior region." *J Periodontol* 72(10): 1364–1371.

Cornelini, R., F. Cangini, et al. (2005). "Immediate restoration of implants placed into fresh extraction sockets for single-tooth replacement: A prospective clinical study." *Int J Periodontics Restorative Dent* 25(5): 439–447.

Dawson, A., S. Chen, et al. (2009). *The SAC Classification in Implant Dentistry*. Berlin: Quintessence.

de Oliveira, R. R., G. O. Macedo, et al. (2009). "Replacement of hopeless retained primary teeth by immediate dental implants: A case report." *Int J Oral Maxillofac Implants* 24(1): 151–154.

Evans, C. D., and S. T. Chen (2008). "Esthetic outcomes of immediate implant placements." *Clin Oral Implants Res* 19(1): 73–80.

Fugazzotto, P. A. (2008a). "Implant placement at the time of mandibular molar extraction: Description of technique and preliminary results of 341 cases." *J Periodontol* 79(4): 737–747.

Fugazzotto, P. A. (2008b). "Implant placement at the time of maxillary molar extraction: Treatment protocols and report of results." *J Periodontol* 79(2): 216–223.

Fugazzotto, P. A., and P. S. De (2002). "Sinus floor augmentation at the time of maxillary molar extraction: Success and failure rates of 137 implants in function for up to 3 years." *J Periodontol* 73(1): 39–44.

Fuss, Z., J. Lustig, et al. (1999). "Prevalence of vertical root fractures in extracted endodontically treated teeth." *Int Endod J* 32(4): 283–286.

Garber, D. A., and U. C. Belser (1995). "Restoration-driven implant placement with restoration-generated site development." *Compend Contin Educ Dent* 16(8): 796, 798–802, 804.

Hammerle, C. H., M. G. Araujo, et al. (2012). "Evidence-based knowledge on the biology and treatment of extraction sockets." *Clin Oral Implants Res* 23 Suppl 5: 80–82.

Hammerle, C. H., P. Stone, et al. (2009). "Consensus statements and recommended clinical procedures regarding computer-assisted implant dentistry." *Int J Oral Maxillofac Implants* 24 Suppl: 126–131.

Kan, J. Y., K. Rungcharassaeng, et al. (2007). "Periimplant tissue response following immediate provisional restoration of scalloped implants in the esthetic zone: A one-year pilot prospective multicenter study." *J Prosthet Dent* 97(6 Suppl): S109–118.

Kan, J. Y., K. Rungcharassaeng, et al. (2003). "Dimensions of peri-implant mucosa: An evaluation of maxillary anterior single implants in humans." *J Periodontol* 74(4): 557–562.

Kois, J. C. (2004). "Predictable single-tooth peri-implant esthetics: Five diagnostic keys." *Compend Contin Educ Dent* 25(11): 895–896, 898, 900 passim; quiz 906–907.

Lazzara, R. J. (1989). "Immediate implant placement into extraction sites: Surgical and restorative advantages." *Int J Periodontics Restorative Dent* 9(5): 332–343.

Mayfield, L., N. Nobreus, et al. (1997). "Guided bone regeneration in dental implant treatment using a bioabsorbable membrane." *Clin Oral Implants Res* 8(1): 10–17.

Norton, M. R. (2004). "A short-term clinical evaluation of immediately restored maxillary TiOblast single-tooth implants." *Int J Oral Maxillofac Implants* 19(2): 274–281.

Rosenberg, E. S., D. A. Garber, et al. (1980). "Tooth lengthening procedures." *Compend Contin Educ Gen Dent* 1(3): 161–172.

Rupprecht, R. D., G. M. Horning, et al. (2001). "Prevalence of dehiscences and fenestrations in modern American skulls." *J Periodontol* 72(6): 722–729.

Ryser, M. R., M. S. Block, et al. (2005). "Correlation of papilla to crestal bone levels around single tooth implants in immediate or delayed crown protocols." *J Oral Maxillofac Surg* 63(8): 1184–1195.

Sabri, R. (1989). "[Crown lengthening by orthodontic extrusion: Principles and techniques]." *J Periodontol* 8(2): 197–204.

Salama, H., and M. Salama (1993). "The role of orthodontic extrusive remodeling in the enhancement of soft and hard tissue profiles prior to implant placement: A systematic approach to the management of extraction site defects." *Int J Periodontics Restorative Dent* 13(4): 312–333.

Wagenberg, B., and S. J. Froum (2006). "A retrospective study of 1925 consecutively placed immediate implants from 1988 to 2004." *Int J Oral Maxillofac Implants* 21(1): 71–80.

Infected Sites

Early in the history of implant dentistry, clinicians recommended a waiting period of 6 months following an extraction prior to the insertion of an endosseous dental implant into the edentulous site (Adell, Lekholm, et al. 1981). As discussed in the chapter on extraction site healing, this waiting period frequently results in a significantly resorbed alveolar process and can influence the ideal positioning of dental implants (Iasella, Greenwell, et al. 2003). The evolution of the immediate placement technique provided a safe and efficient method of treatment that eliminated the 6-month waiting period, maintained the alveolar housing, decreased surgical time and procedures, reduced cost and improved acceptance for the patient, and potentially provided better axial alignment, esthetics, and biomechanical prosthetics (Lazzara 1989; Parel and Triplett 1990; Shanaman 1992; Werbitt and Goldberg 1992; Schultz 1993; Watzek, Haider, et al. 1995; Missika, Abbou, et al. 1997). Despite these advantages, immediate implant placement may

be considered to have several contraindications. These perceived contraindications include intimate contact to anatomical structures such as the mandibular canal, maxillary sinuses, or nasal cavity; bone loss to the root apex; inability to obtain primary stability or primary flap closure; and the presence of periodontal disease, periapical lesions, or purulent exudate (Block and Kent 1990; Wilson 1992; Arlin 1993; Rosenquist and Grenthe 1996; Grunder, Polizzi, et al. 1999; Polizzi, Grunder, et al. 2000). This last consideration, the question of whether or not an infected site contraindicates immediate implant placement, has engendered the most controversy and remains an ongoing discussion in the literature today.

Most recently, Chen and colleagues published a report classifying implant placement protocol based on morphological, dimensional, and histologic changes that occur following tooth loss (Table 4.1) (Chen, Wilson, et al. 2004). Each classification type from I to IV offers advantages and disadvantages to treatment

Surgical Essentials of Immediate Implant Dentistry, First Edition. Jay R. Beagle.
© 2013 John Wiley & Sons, Inc. Published 2013 by John Wiley & Sons, Inc.

Table 4.1   Implant timing classification table.

Class	Definition	Advantages	Disadvantages
Type I	Implant placement as part of the same surgical procedure and *immediately* following tooth extraction	Reduced number of surgical procedures Reduced overall treatment time Optimal availability of existing bone	Site morphology may complicate optimal placement and anchorage Thin tissue phenotype may compromise optimal outcome Potential lack of keratinized mucosa for flap adaptation Adjunctive surgical procedures may be required *Technique-sensitive procedure*
Type II	*Complete soft tissue coverage* of the socket (4–8 weeks)	Increased soft tissue area and volume facilitates soft tissue flap management Allows assessment of resolution of local pathology	Site morphology may complicate optimal placement and anchorage Increased treatment time Varying amounts of resorption of the socket walls Adjunctive surgical procedures may be required *Technique-sensitive procedure*
Type III	*Substantial bone fill* of the socket (12–16 weeks)	Substantial bone fill of the socket facilitates implant placement Mature soft tissues facilitate flap management	Increased treatment time Adjunctive surgical procedures may be required Varying amounts of resorption of the socket walls
Type IV	*Healed site* (>6 months)	Clinically healed ridge Mature soft tissues facilitate flap management	Increased treatment time Adjunctive surgical procedures may be required Large variation in available bone volume

From Chen, Wilson, et al. 2004. Courtesy of Quintessence Publishing.

timing, with the evaluation of the site to ultimately be critical in the determination of treatment modalities. One significant aspect of placement timing with this classification system concerned the presence of infection at the time of tooth extraction. It was concluded that the T-1 approach (immediate placement) should not be utilized in the presence of infection. Rather, these authors recommended that the surgeon select a T-2 (early) or T-3 (delayed) protocol to achieve a more predictable outcome. This, Chen and colleagues argued, posed less risk regarding both osseointegration and ideal esthetic outcome.

The placement of immediate dental implants in the presence of a periapical or periodontal infection has been contraindicated by other authors as well. Notably, these publications primarily focus their argument on human case reports (Lundgren and Nyman 1991; Tolman and Keller 1991; Werbitt and Goldberg 1992; Rosenquist and Grenthe 1996; Grunder, Polizzi, et al. 1999; Rosenberg, Cho, et al. 2004; Wagenberg and Froum 2006). Also of note, these studies utilized machine-screw implants and ePTFE membranes, while showing a lower success rate and higher incidence of post-operative infections.

Contrary to these reports, others have shown both with animal studies and human trials that experimentally induced periodontal or periapical lesions did not affect the ability for implants to predictably osseointegrate (Table 4.2) (Novaes and Novaes 1995; Novaes, Vidigal, et al. 1998; Marcaccini, Novaes, et al. 2003; Novaes, Marcaccini, et al. 2003; Novaes, Papalexiou, et al. 2004; Papalexiou, Novaes, et al. 2004). Case reports as well as prospective randomized controlled studies in humans with periapical lesions have shown success rates of 92–100%. Siegentholer et al. treated seventeen patients consecutively having periapical lesions using immediately placed roughened surface implants (Siegenthaler, Jung, et al. 2007). In this study, GBR using deproteinized bovine bone and a resorbable collagen membrane was utilized in treating the apical fenestrations and HDD. All implants were loaded at 3 months and observed for 12 months with a 100% success rate. These authors concluded that a critical aspect of the treatment was assessing the diameter of the periapical lesion. If the lesion exceeded the diameter of the planned implant, then there was a need to obtain primary stability in an apical direction. In these situations, the use of CT diagnostics to view the root morphology and osseous lesion may assist the clinician in treatment planning for either an immediate or delayed placement protocol.

A series of animal studies involving the placement of immediate implants in the dog model with periodontal disease also indicated that chronic infection should not be a contraindication for this treatment method. In one study reported by Novaes et al. (2003), five dogs were treated using a split mouth design in which one quadrant served as a control, and the other quadrant underwent ligature-induced periodontitis. After 3 months, the mandibular premolars were removed in both sites, and implants having a roughened surface were immediately placed. The animals were sacrificed after a healing period of 12 weeks, and the specimens were analyzed histologically. Both test and control groups showed good bone-to-implant contact with a percentage of 66% and 62.4%, respectively. This difference was found to be statistically insignificant. The authors concluded that periodontally infected sites may not be a contraindication for immediate dental implants if adequate pre- and post-operative care is taken, such as the use of broad spectrum antibiotics, thorough plaque control, achievement of primary stability, and the selection of appropriate biomaterials.

SUMMARY

A significant quantity of literature has been published pertaining to the placement of immediate dental implants; however, there is a paucity of peer-reviewed articles, by comparison, related to immediately placed dental implants into infected sites. Nearly all reports contraindicating this technique are human case reports that have employed similar treatment modalities, namely machined implant surfaces and ePTFE membranes. By today's standards, both of these biomaterials are considered outdated, having been replaced with roughened surfaced implants and bioresorbable membranes posing less risk to the patient, increased predictability, and fewer complications. A number of evidence-based animal and human studies indicate immediate implants having a roughened surface and utilizing collagen membranes when necessary, placed in extraction sockets exhibiting either periodontal or periapical lesions, do not lead to an increased rate of complications and can have similar success rates as those placed in non-infected areas. Of primary concern is the ability to achieve primary mechanical stability at the time of placement by engaging bone apically or along the lateral walls of the extraction site. Treatment planning for immediately placed dental implants in infected sites should assess esthetic risk factors as described by Morton et al. to minimize or prevent unfavorable

Table 4.2 Infected site immediate placement.

Author	N	Periapical/ Periodontal	Human/Animal	Surface	Membrane	Survival
Lundgren et al. 1991	1	Both	Human	Machine	ePTFE	100%
Wilson 1992	4	Both	Human	Machine/HA	ePTFE	25%
Werbitt et al. 1992	8	Both	Human	Machine	ePTFE	100%
Novaes et al. 1995	3	Periapical	Human	HA	Cellulose	100%
Pecora et al. 1996	32	Periapical	Human	Machine	None	98%
Novaes et al. 1998	15	Periapical	Animal	TPS	None	100%
Grunder et al. 1999	113	Both	Human	Machine	None	89.8%
Papalexiou et al. 2004	36	Periodontal	Animal	SLA/TPS	None	100%
Marcaccini et al. 2003	40	Periodontal	Animal	SLA	None	100%
Novaes et al. 2003	40	Periodontal	Animal	SLA	None	100%
Novaes et al. 2003	36	Periodontal	Animal	SLA	None	100%
Marcaccini et al. 2003	40	Periodontal	Animal	SLA	None	100%

outcomes (Morton, Martin, et al. 2004). The availability of CT radiography may offer the clinician greater insight to treatment planning these cases for immediate versus delayed placement especially in situations where the ability to achieve primary stability is in question (Figures 4.1–4.62).

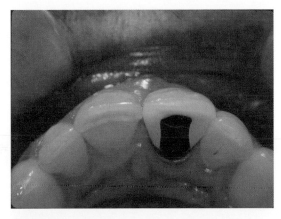

Figure 4.3   Occlusal view pre-op tooth #9.

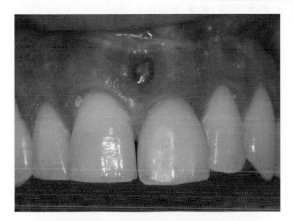

Figure 4.1   Buccal view pre-op tooth #9—note fistula.

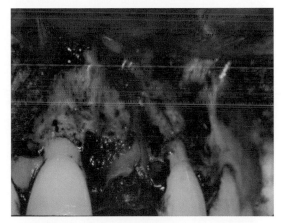

Figure 4.4   Buccal view tooth #9 before extraction—note vertical root fracture.

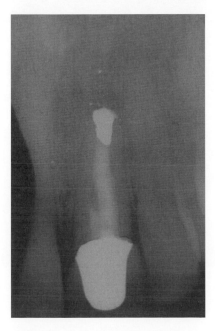

Figure 4.2   Pre-op radiograph tooth #9.

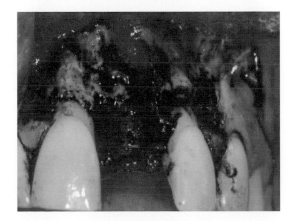

Figure 4.5   Buccal view tooth #9 following extraction.

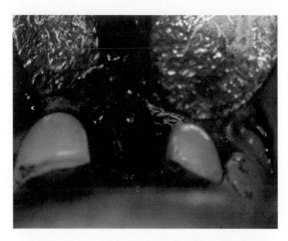

Figure 4.6 Occlusal view tooth #9 following extraction.

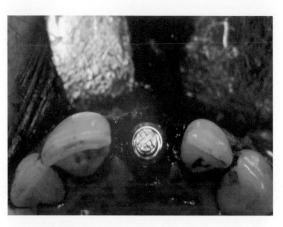

Figure 4.8 Occlusal view of tooth #9 implant following placement.

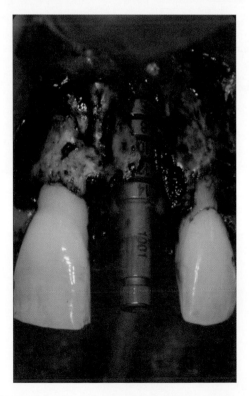

Figure 4.7 Buccal view of completed osteotomy.

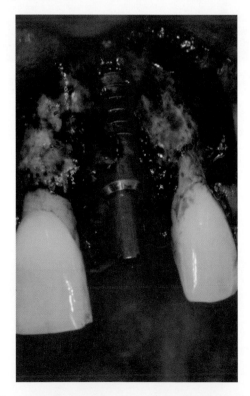

Figure 4.9 Buccal view of tooth #9 implant following placement.

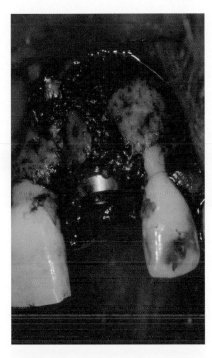

Figure 4.10 Autogenous bone graft placed over buccal dehiscence.

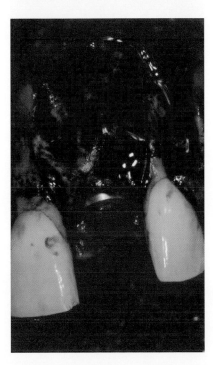

Figure 4.11 Resorbable membrane positioned over autogenous bone graft.

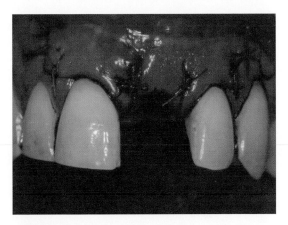

Figure 4.12 Buccal view of a semi-submerged flap closure.

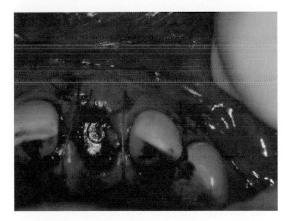

Figure 4.13 Occlusal view of semi-submerged flap closure.

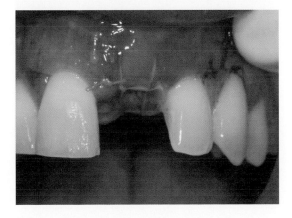

Figure 4.14 Buccal view of 2-week post-op.

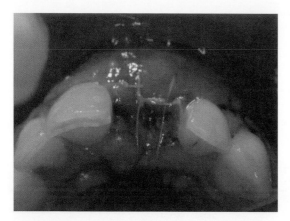

Figure 4.15   Occlusal view of 2-week post-op.

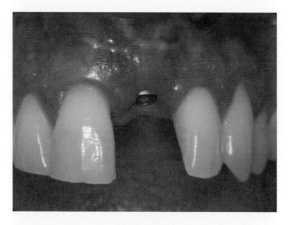

Figure 4.16   Buccal view of 12-week post-op.

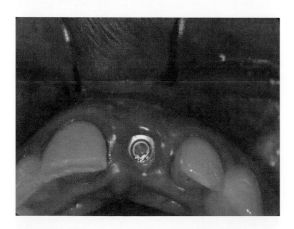

Figure 4.17   Occlusal view of 12-week post-op.

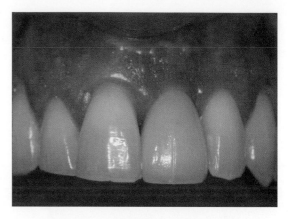

Figure 4.18   Final restoration of tooth #9 treated with immediate placement.

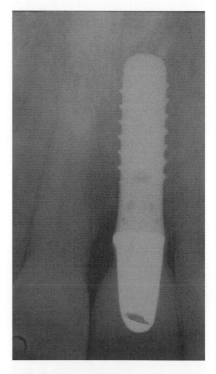

Figure 4.19   Final radiograph of tooth #9 treated with immediate placement.

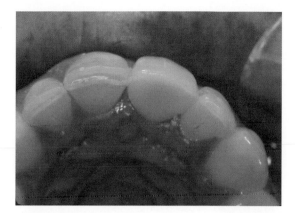

Figure 4.20 Occlusal view of final restoration for tooth #9.

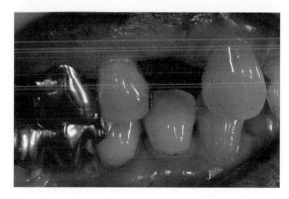

Figure 4.21 Pre-op buccal view of teeth #3–6.

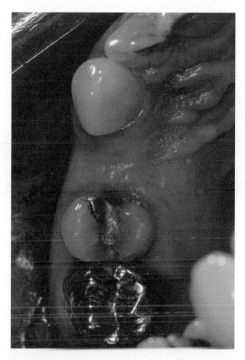

Figure 4.22 Pre-op occlusal view of teeth #3–6.

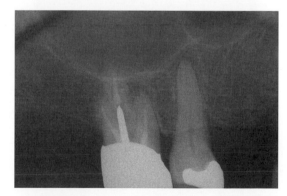

Figure 4.23 Pre-op radiograph of teeth #3 and #4. Note periapical lesions on the mesial buccal root of #3 and the apex of #4.

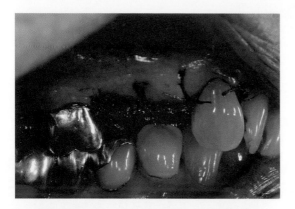

Figure 4.24   Buccal view of flap closure following the mesial buccal root resection of tooth #3, type I implant placement for tooth #4, and type IV implant placement for tooth #5.

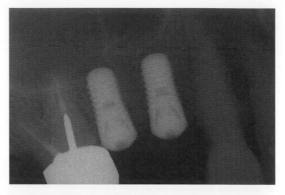

Figure 4.26   Post-op radiograph of teeth #3–6.

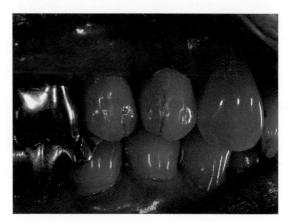

Figure 4.27   Buccal view of final restoration for teeth #4 and #5.

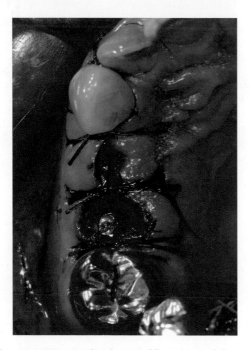

Figure 4.25   Occlusal view of flap closure following the mesial buccal root resection of tooth #3, type I implant placement for tooth #4, and type IV implant placement for tooth #5.

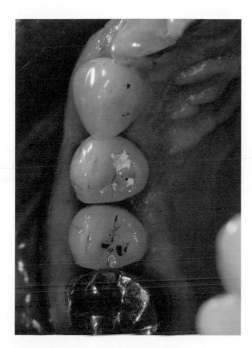

Figure 4.28 Occlusal view of final restoration for teeth #4 and #5.

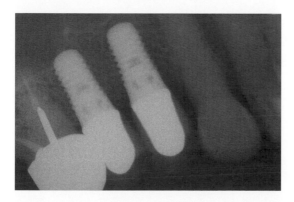

Figure 4.29 Final radiograph of teeth #3–6.

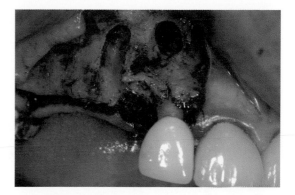

Figure 4.30 Buccal view of surgical site involving the extraction of tooth #6 due to a vertical root fracture.

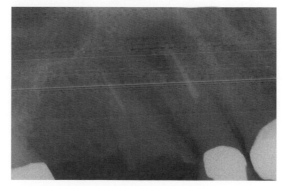

Figure 4.31 Pre-op radiograph of teeth #3–8.

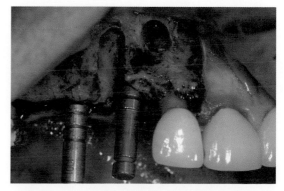

Figure 4.32 Buccal view of osteotomies for type IV placement for tooth #5 and type I placement for tooth #6.

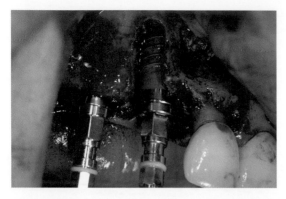

Figure 4.33 Buccal view of implant placement for teeth #5 and #6.

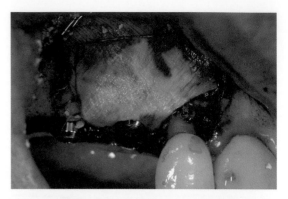

Figure 4.36 Placement of a resorbable membrane over the osseous grafts.

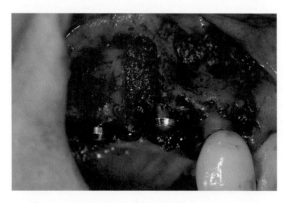

Figure 4.34 Treatment of the dehiscence of periapical osseous lesions with autogenous bone graft.

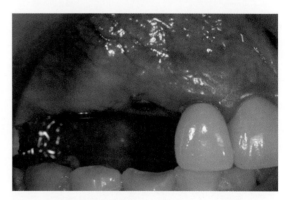

Figure 4.37 Buccal view of the surgical site following 12 weeks of healing.

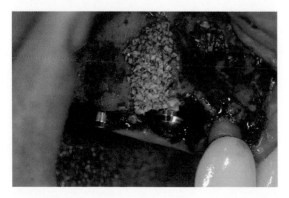

Figure 4.35 Addition of a xenograft veneer over the autogenous bone graft.

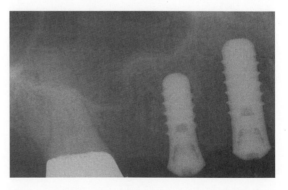

Figure 4.38 12-week post-op radiograph.

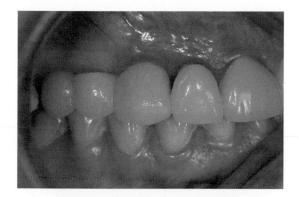

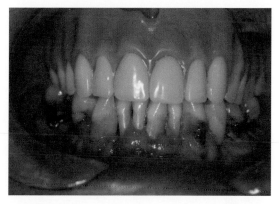

Figure 4.39 Final restoration with teeth #5 and #6 splinted and tooth #4 cantilevered.

Figure 4.41 Pre-op buccal view of mandibular dentition having advanced periodontal disease and recurrent root caries.

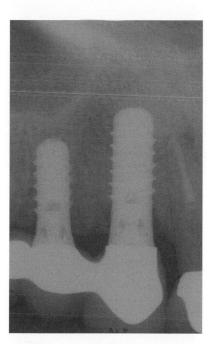

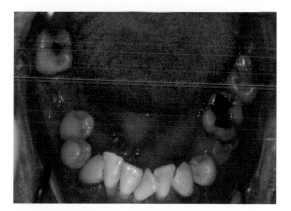

Figure 4.42 Pre-op occlusal view of mandibular dentition having advanced periodontal disease and recurrent root caries.

Figure 4.40 Final radiograph of teeth #5–7.

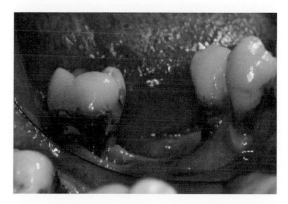

Figure 4.43 Pre-op of right posterior buccal view of mandibular dentition having advanced periodontal disease and recurrent root caries.

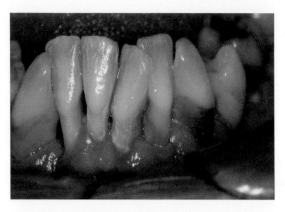

Figure 4.44 Pre-op of anterior buccal view of mandibular dentition having advanced periodontal disease and recurrent root caries.

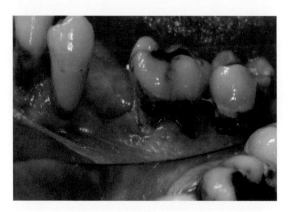

Figure 4.45 Pre-op of left posterior buccal view of mandibular dentition having advanced periodontal disease and recurrent root caries.

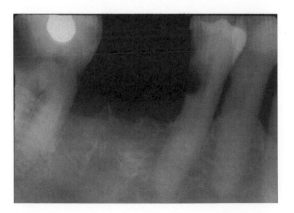

Figure 4.46 Pre-op radiograph of teeth #28–31.

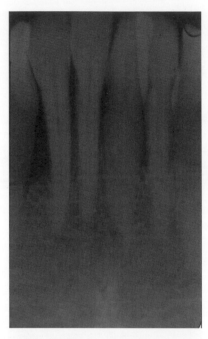

Figure 4.47 Pre-op radiograph of teeth #24–27.

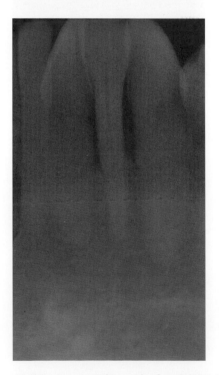

Figure 4.48 Pre-op radiograph of teeth #22–25.

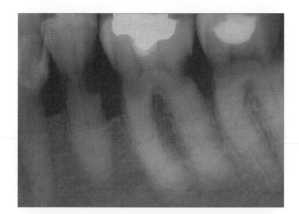

Figure 4.49 Pre-op radiograph of teeth #18–21.

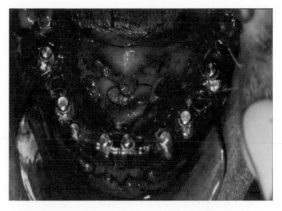

Figure 4.52 Occlusal view of immediate implant placement with surgical stent in place.

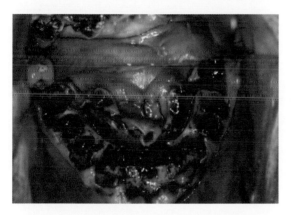

Figure 4.50 Occlusal view of extraction sites.

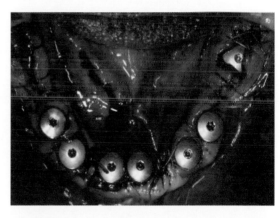

Figure 4.53 Occlusal view of flap closure following immediate implant placement. Note tooth #30 healing abutment fully submerged due to limited primary stability.

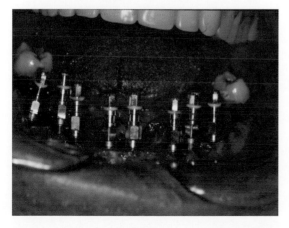

Figure 4.51 Buccal view of immediate implant placement.

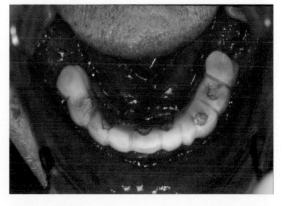

Figure 4.54 Occlusal view of immediate load fixed provisional bridge.

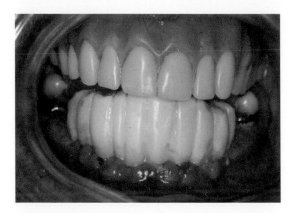

Figure 4.55 Buccal view of immediate load fixed provisional bridge.

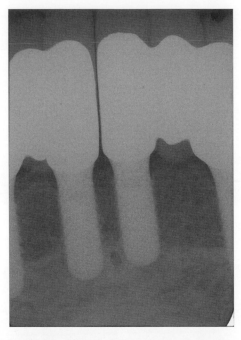

Figure 4.57 Final radiograph of teeth #22–27.

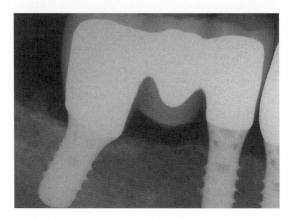

Figure 4.56 Final radiograph of teeth #28–30.

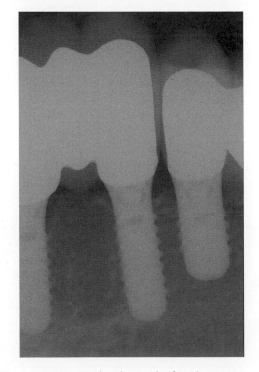

Figure 4.58 Final radiograph of teeth #21–24.

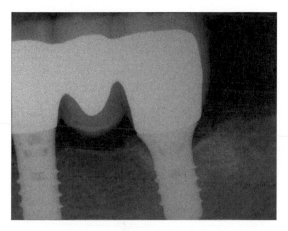

Figure 4.59   Final radiograph of teeth #19–21.

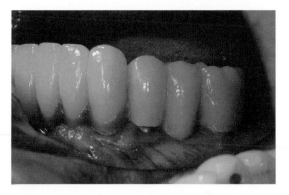

Figure 4.62   Buccal view of final restoration of teeth #19–24.

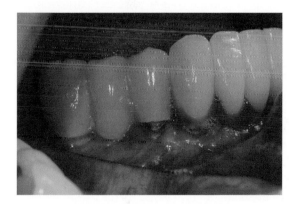

Figure 4.60   Buccal view of final restorations for teeth #25–30.

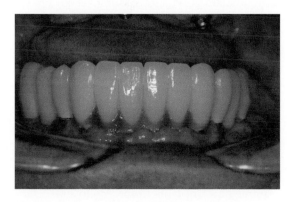

Figure 4.61   Buccal view of final restoration.

References

Adell, R., U. Lekholm, et al. (1981). "A 15-year study of osseointegrated implants in the treatment of the edentulous jaw." *Int J Oral Surg* 10(6): 387–416.

Arlin, M. (1993). "Immediate placement of dental implants into extraction sockets: Surgically-related difficulties." *Oral Health* 83(7): 23–24, 27–28, 31 passim.

Block, M. S., and J. N. Kent (1990). "Factors associated with soft- and hard-tissue compromise of endosseous implants." *J Oral Maxillofac Surg* 48(11): 1153–1160.

Chen, S. T., T. G. Wilson, Jr., et al. (2004). "Immediate or early placement of implants following tooth extraction: Review of biologic basis, clinical procedures, and outcomes." *Int J Oral Maxillofac Implants* 19 Suppl: 12–25.

Grunder, U., G. Polizzi, et al. (1999). "A 3-year prospective multicenter follow-up report on the immediate and delayed-immediate placement of implants." *Int J Oral Maxillofac Implants* 14(2): 210–216.

Iasella, J. M., H. Greenwell, et al. (2003). "Ridge preservation with freeze-dried bone allograft and a collagen membrane compared to extraction alone for implant site development: A clinical and histologic study in humans." *J Periodontol* 74(7): 990–999.

Lazzara, R. J. (1989). "Immediate implant placement into extraction sites: Surgical and restorative advantages." *Int J Periodontics Restorative Dent* 9(5): 332–343.

Lundgren, D., and S. Nyman (1991). "Bone regeneration in 2 stages for retention of dental implant: A case report." *Clin Oral Implants Res* 2(4): 203–207.

Marcaccini, A. M., A. B. Novaes, Jr., et al. (2003). "Immediate placement of implants into periodontally infected sites in dogs. Part 2: A fluorescence microscopy study." *Int J Oral Maxillofac Implants* 18(6): 812–819.

Missika, P., M. Abbou, et al. (1997). "Osseous regeneration in immediate postextraction implant placement: A literature review and clinical evaluation." *Pract Periodontics Aesthet Dent* 9(2): 165–175; quiz 176.

Morton, D., W. C. Martin, et al. (2004). "Single-stage Straumann dental implants in the aesthetic zone: Considerations and treatment procedures." *J Oral Maxillofac Surg* 62(9 Suppl 2): 57–66.

Novaes, A. B., Jr., A. M. Marcaccini, et al. (2003). "Immediate placement of implants into periodontally infected sites in dogs: A histomorphometric study of bone-implant contact." *Int J Oral Maxillofac Implants* 18(3): 391–398.

Novaes, A. B., Jr., and A. B. Novaes (1995). "Immediate implants placed into infected sites: A clinical report." *Int J Oral Maxillofac Implants* 10(5): 609–613.

Novaes, A. B., Jr., V. Papalexiou, et al. (2004). "Influence of implant microstructure on the osseointegration of immediate implants placed in periodontally infected sites: A histomorphometric study in dogs." *Clin Oral Implants Res* 15(1): 34–43.

Novaes, A. B., Jr., G. M. Vidigal, Jr., et al. (1998). "Immediate implants placed into infected sites: A histomorphometric study in dogs." *Int J Oral Maxillofac Implants* 13(3): 422–427.

Papalexiou, V., A. B. Novaes, Jr., et al. (2004). "Influence of implant microstructure on the dynamics of bone healing around immediate implants placed into periodontally infected

sites: A confocal laser scanning microscopic study." *Clin Oral Implants Res* 15(1): 44–53.

Parel, S. M., and R. G. Triplett (1990). "Immediate fixture placement: A treatment planning alternative." *Int J Oral Maxillofac Implants* 5(4): 337–345.

Pecora, G., S. Andreana, et al. (1996). "New directions in surgical endodontics: Immediate implantation into an extraction site." *J Endod* 22(3): 135–139.

Polizzi, G., U. Grunder, et al. (2000). "Immediate and delayed implant placement into extraction sockets: A 5-year report." *Clin Implant Dent Relat Res* 2(2): 93–99.

Rosenberg, E. S., S. C. Cho, et al. (2004). "A comparison of characteristics of implant failure and survival in periodontally compromised and periodontally healthy patients: A clinical report." *Int J Oral Maxillofac Implants* 19(6): 873–879.

Rosenquist, B., and B. Grenthe (1996). "Immediate placement of implants into extraction sockets: Implant survival." *Int J Oral Maxillofac Implants* 11(2): 205–209.

Schultz, A. J. (1993). "Guided tissue regeneration (GTR) of nonsubmerged implants in immediate extraction sites." *Pract Periodontics Aesthet Dent* 5(2): 59–65; quiz 66.

Shanaman, R. H. (1992). "The use of guided tissue regeneration to facilitate ideal prosthetic placement of implants." *Int J Periodontics Restorative Dent* 12(4): 256–265.

Siegenthaler, D. W., R. E. Jung, et al. (2007). "Replacement of teeth exhibiting periapical pathology by immediate implants: A prospective, controlled clinical trial." *Clin Oral Implants Res* 18(6): 727–737.

Tolman, D. E., and E. E. Keller (1991). "Endosseous implant placement immediately following dental extraction and alveoloplasty: Preliminary report with 6-year follow-up." *Int J Oral Maxillofac Implants* 6(1): 24–28.

Wagenberg, B., and S. J. Froum (2006). "A retrospective study of 1925 consecutively placed immediate implants from 1988 to 2004." *Int J Oral Maxillofac Implants* 21(1): 71–80.

Watzek, G., R. Haider, et al. (1995). "Immediate and delayed implantation for complete restoration of the jaw following extraction of all residual teeth: A retrospective study comparing different types of serial immediate implantation." *Int J Oral Maxillofac Implants* 10(5): 561–567.

Werbitt, M. J., and P. V. Goldberg (1992). "The immediate implant: Bone preservation and bone regeneration." *Int J Periodontics Restorative Dent* 12(3): 206–217.

Wilson, T. G., Jr. (1992). "Guided tissue regeneration around dental implants in immediate and recent extraction sites: Initial observations." *Int J Periodontics Restorative Dent* 12(3): 185–193.

Extraction Site Healing **5**

Clinicians who embark on the reconstruction of partially and fully edentulous patients utilizing dental implants must have a thorough understanding of wound healing following the loss of a tooth. It is widely accepted that a three-dimensional alteration of the bone and associated soft tissues occurs following a tooth extraction (Carlsson, Bergman, et al. 1967; Atwood and Coy 1971). This finding implies that the replacement of the lost root with an endosseous dental implant may result in a non-desirable functional or esthetic outcome if the bone architecture is not properly evaluated prior to implant surgery (Figures 5.1 and 5.2) (Iasella, Greenwell, et al. 2003). Knowledge concerning the stages of wound healing following an extraction will help guide the surgeon in the necessary critical thinking required when determining if a site should be treated using an immediate, early, or delayed implant approach (Chen, Wilson, et al. 2004). With this

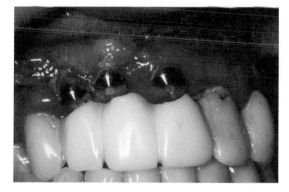

Figure 5.1 Buccal view of poor implant placement due to inadequate bone architecture.

end in mind, numerous "classic" articles have been published using animal research and human biopsies to create a scaffold of knowledge regarding wound healing, bone resorption, regeneration, and remodeling of the extraction socket.

Surgical Essentials of Immediate Implant Dentistry, First Edition. Jay R. Beagle.
© 2013 John Wiley & Sons, Inc. Published 2013 by John Wiley & Sons, Inc.

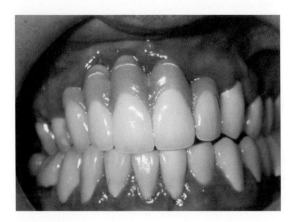

Figure 5.2 Buccal view of final restoration of implants placed into sites with inadequate bone architecture.

ANIMAL STUDIES

Much of the detailed information regarding wound healing has been derived from animal studies. Animal studies provide us an opportunity to histologically assess a mathematical "time lapse" sequence of events not possible to control with humans. Quite often, these studies provide a control to compare to sites deemed experimental. The control sites typically allow for an unblemished extraction socket to compare to one treated with a bone graft and/or dental implant. An assessment of the literature shows a rather consistent outcome of the histological events that occur following tooth extraction, particularly in the dog model (Cardaropoli, Wennstrom, et al. 2003; Araujo and Lindhe 2005). Following the extraction of a tooth, five stages of healing occur (Amler, Johnson, et al. 1960). Initially, a blood clot forms as a coagulum of red and white blood cells, derived from the circulation. During the second stage, the clot is replaced over a 4- to 5-day period with granulation tissue. During this time, endothelial cells are associated with budding capillaries. From days 14 to 16, the third stage consists of the granulation tissue being replaced by connective tissue. Spindle-shaped fibroblasts,

collagen fibers, and a metachromatic ground substance comprise the connective tissue.

Osteoid calcification commences at the apex and lateral walls of the socket during the fourth stage of healing, seen within an additional 7–10 days. By the sixth week, the socket is almost completely filled by bone trabeculae. During this time, maximum osteoblastic activity is occurring but subsides after the eighth week. The fifth stage is characterized by the completion of epithelial closure of the socket, occurring between 24 and 35 days. From weeks 5 to 10, substantial bone fill occurs, being completed at week 16.

Animal studies have also given us insight into the histologic events that occur as the internal and external dimensions of the socket change during wound healing. The information extrapolated from this data has a direct correlation to treatment planning of dental implants, especially relative to the desired prosthetic result compared to implant position. These dimensional changes occurring in the dog model for extraction sites have been described with regards to rate and dimensional direction through histologic observations (Araujo and Lindhe 2005; Araujo, Sukekava, et al. 2006). During the first week of healing, the marginal portion of the lingual boney wall of the socket is markedly wider than the buccal wall (Figure 5.3). Both walls contain large numbers of well-defined bone marrow spaces, with the inner surfaces of the socket walls lined with bundle bone. It has been observed that at week 1, the buccal bone crest is made exclusively of bundle bone, while the lingual crest is comprised of a mixture of cortical bone and bundle bone. During this time, the height of the buccal wall is more pronounced than that of the lingual plate by >1 mm. Histologically, large numbers of osteoclasts are observed along the outer surface of the buccal and lingual crest walls. Also during week 1, the internal portion of the extraction socket is comprised of coagulum, granulation tissues, provisional matrix, and small amounts of newly formed bone, seen in the most apical portion of the socket. At this time sequence, the provisional matrix is the

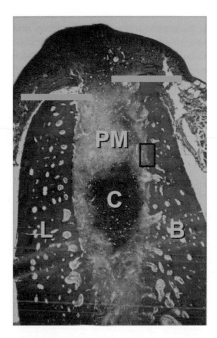

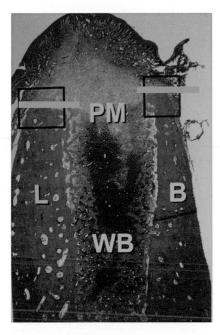

Figure 5.3 Histology showing 1 week of healing. Reprinted from Araujo, M. G., and J. Lindhe (2005). "Dimensional ridge alterations following tooth extraction: An experimental study in the dog." *J Clin Periodontol* 32(2): 212–218, with permission from John Wiley & Sons, Inc.

Figure 5.4 Histology showing 2 weeks of healing. Reprinted from Araujo, M. G., and J. Lindhe (2005). "Dimensional ridge alterations following tooth extraction: An experimental study in the dog." *J Clin Periodontol* 32(2): 212–218, with permission from John Wiley & Sons, Inc.

dominant tissue, consisting of fibroblasts, new vessels, and collagen fibers.

During the second week of wound healing, the crestal region of the lingual bone wall is absent of bundle bone, while the corresponding region of the buccal bone wall continues to have bundle bone present (Figure 5.4). Osteoclasts continue to be observed in the crestal region of both bone walls, as well as areas apical to the crest. As large amounts of newly formed bone are noted in the apical and lateral aspects of the socket, the provisional matrix continues to survive in the central and marginal compartments. The second week is also noted for the absence of the periodontal ligament. The remaining bundle bone is seen in direct continuity of the woven bone, lined with osteoblasts and a primitive bone marrow.

By week 4, bundle bone is also found to be vacant from the buccal bone wall (Figure 5.5).

The lamellar bone of the buccal wall is replaced by woven bone, exhibiting signs of remodeling via the presence of osteoclasts. The lingual and buccal walls are also observed to be narrower than at week 1, both at the crest and mid-root levels. The provisional matrix now occupies only the most central portion of the healing socket while the remainder of the socket area is comprised of mineralized tissue and bone marrow. This mineralized tissue, mainly comprised as woven bone, is in a state of both modeling and remodeling.

At the eighth week following tooth extraction, the lingual bone wall is dimensionally wider than the corresponding buccal bone wall (Figure 5.6). The buccal bone wall is also consistently located about 2mm apical to the height of the lingual crestal bone. The buccal and lingual walls are observed to have a mineralized "bridge" consisting of woven and

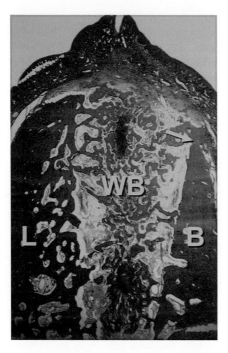

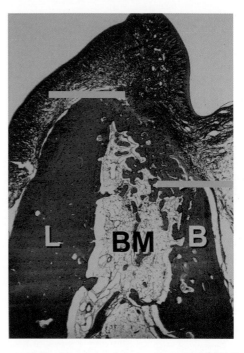

Figure 5.5 Histology showing 4 weeks of healing. Reprinted from Araujo, M. G., and J. Lindhe (2005). "Dimensional ridge alterations following tooth extraction: An experimental study in the dog." *J Clin Periodontol* 32(2): 212–218, with permission from John Wiley & Sons, Inc.

Figure 5.6 Histology showing 8 weeks of healing. Reprinted from Araujo, M. G., and J. Lindhe (2005). "Dimensional ridge alterations following tooth extraction: An experimental study in the dog." *J Clin Periodontol* 32(2): 212–218, with permission from John Wiley & Sons, Inc.

lamellar bone. The outer surfaces of both buccal and lingual walls are observed as having scattered osteoclasts extending from the crest to the apical portion of the socket. Bone marrow is now the predominant tissue found in the internal portion of the socket with few trabeculae of woven and lamellar bone present.

These observations noted during the 8-week study of the extraction socket in the dog model confirm histologically the dimensional changes observed internally and externally during wound healing. As a result of osteoclastic activity and loss of bundle bone, the width and height of the buccal and lingual bone walls is found to be reduced, with the most pronounced change occurring with the dimensions of the buccal wall.

Further study in the process of bone resorption following extraction is still needed with the animal model. Future observations may

provide answers to the importance of bundle bone, the effect of elevating a full-thickness muccoperiosteal flap for extractions, the adaptation to the continued lack of function at the extraction site, and the tissue adjustment to meet "genetically" determined demands regarding the ridge geometry with the loss of teeth (Fickl, Zuhr, et al. 2008; Araujo and Lindhe 2009).

HUMAN STUDIES

The challenge of developing a well-controlled human histologic study following the extraction of teeth is evident by the paucity of scientific literature on the subject (Van der Weijden, Dell'Acqua, et al. 2009). Fortunately, those studies reported follow the sequence of events observed in the dog model (Araujo and

Lindhe 2005; Araujo, Sukekava, et al. 2006; Araujo and Lindhe 2009). More often discussed in the literature are the morphologic changes of the external dimensions of the extraction socket in humans. These findings are based on cephalometric measurements, study cast measurements, subtraction radiography, and direct measurements of the ridge following surgical re-entry procedures (Schropp, Wenzel, et al. 2003). Using radiographic cephalographs, both Atwood et al. and Carlsson et al. have observed the height and width changes occurring with the edentulous maxilla and mandible following tooth extraction (Carlsson, Bergman, et al. 1967; Atwood and Coy 1971). Carlsson's observations were made over a 5-year timeline for patients who had received immediate dentures.

Studies by Johnson and by Lekovic et al. have reported on the alveolar changes occurring following tooth loss using measurements from diagnostic study casts (Johnson 1963; Johnson 1969; Lekovic, Kenney, et al. 1997). The changes observed reflect both the alterations of dimensions in the hard tissues and overlying soft tissue mucosa. During the initial 6- to 12-month period, 5–7 mm of horizontal reduction occurs, representing approximately 50% of the initial ridge width. Also noted in this time frame is a corresponding resorption of vertical height ranging from 2.0 to 4.5 mm. Of interest is that greater vertical dimensional changes seem to occur with multiple adjacent extractions compared to single sites.

The classic paper by Schropp and co-workers utilized subtraction radiography and study cast measurements when observing forty-six healing sockets in forty-six patients followed for 4–12 months (Schropp, Wenzel, et al. 2003). The extraction sites observed involved both maxillary and mandibular molars and premolars. The authors reported a reduction in buccal lingual width of approximately 50% (from 12.0 mm to 5.9 mm) over the 12-month study period, with 66% of this change developing within the first 12 weeks of healing. Also noted after 3 months post-extraction was a loss of buccal crest height measuring 0.8 mm. Based on

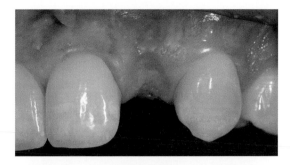

Figure 5.7 Buccal view of pre-op type III implant placed for tooth #10.

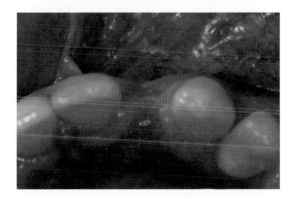

Figure 5.8 Occlusal view of pre-op type III implant placed for tooth #10.

this report, it is suggested that if an implant is planned for a site, it should be placed as soon as possible following an extraction to provide an ideal prosthetic outcome relative to implant positioning, as a delay in treating an edentulous site with an implant will increase the probability of the need for bone augmentation, either simultaneously or prior to implant placement.

The clinician must be observant that the healing potential of the extraction site in patients may differ from what is observed in controlled animal and human studies. A variety of systemic factors (patient's general health and habits) and local factors (number and proximity of teeth to be extracted, pre- and post-operative condition of the socket, tissue phenotypes, and interim prostheses) may influence the rate and degree of alveolar changes (Figures 5.7–5.18) (Chen, Wilson, et al. 2004). Of interest for continued

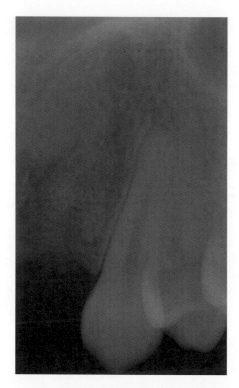

Figure 5.9 Pre-op radiograph for type III implant placement for tooth #10.

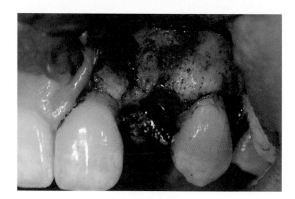

Figure 5.10 Buccal view of tooth #10 surgical site.

research are the effect of post-extraction bone grafting, the use of growth factors and bone morphogenic proteins, the use of barrier membranes, and immediate implant placement with and without immediate loading.

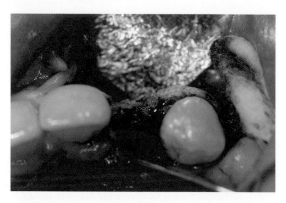

Figure 5.11 Occlusal view of tooth #10 surgical site.

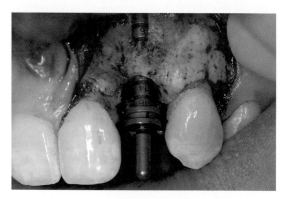

Figure 5.12 Buccal view of tooth #10 implant following osteotomy preparation and fenestration.

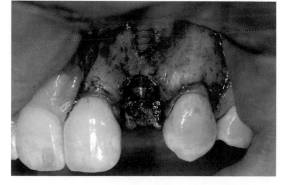

Figure 5.13 Buccal view of tooth #10 implant placement.

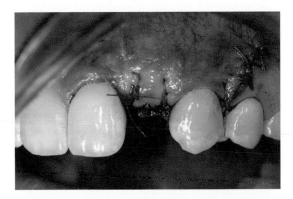

Figure 5.14 Buccal view of semi-submerged flap closure for tooth #10.

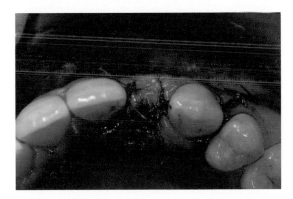

Figure 5.15 Occlusal view of semi-submerged flap closure for tooth #10.

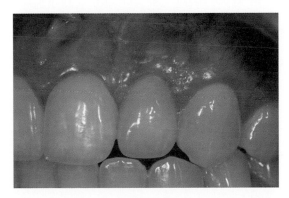

Figure 5.16 Final restoration of type III implant placed for tooth #10.

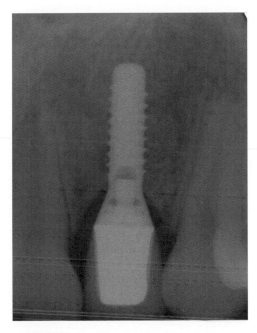

Figure 5.17 Final radiograph of type III implant placed for tooth #10.

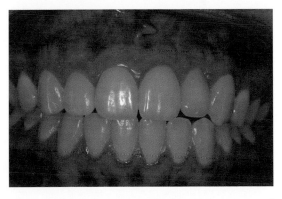

Figure 5.18 Buccal view of gingival asymmetry of implant restoration for tooth #10.

References

Amler, M. H., P. L. Johnson, et al. (1960). "Histological and histochemical investigation of human alveolar socket healing in undisturbed extraction wounds." *J Am Dent Assoc* 61: 32–44.

Araujo, M. G., and J. Lindhe (2005). "Dimensional ridge alterations following tooth extraction: An experimental study in the dog." *J Clin Periodontol* 32(2): 212–218.

Araujo, M. G., and J. Lindhe (2009). "Ridge alterations following tooth extraction with and without flap elevation: An experimental study in the dog." *Clin Oral Implants Res* 20(6): 545–549.

Araujo, M. G., F. Sukekava, et al. (2006). "Tissue modeling following implant placement in fresh extraction sockets." *Clin Oral Implants Res* 17(6): 615–624.

Atwood, D. A., and W. A. Coy (1971). "Clinical, cephalometric, and densitometric study of reduction of residual ridges." *J Prosthet Dent* 26(3): 280–295.

Cardaropoli, G., J. L. Wennstrom, et al. (2003). "Peri-implant bone alterations in relation to inter-unit distances: A 3-year retrospective study." *Clin Oral Implants Res* 14(4): 430–436.

Carlsson, G. E., B. Bergman, et al. (1967). "Changes in contour of the maxillary alveolar process under immediate dentures: A longitudinal clinical and x-ray cephalometric study covering 5 years." *Acta Odontol Scand* 25(1): 45–75.

Chen, S. T., T. G. Wilson, Jr., et al. (2004). "Immediate or early placement of implants following tooth extraction: Review of biologic basis, clinical procedures, and outcomes." *Int J Oral Maxillofac Implants* 19 Suppl: 12–25.

Fickl, S., O. Zuhr, et al. (2008). "Dimensional changes of the alveolar ridge contour after different socket preservation techniques." *J Clin Periodontol* 35: 906–913.

Iasella, J. M., H. Greenwell, et al. (2003). "Ridge preservation with freeze-dried bone allograft and a collagen membrane compared to extraction alone for implant site development: A clinical and histologic study in humans." *J Periodontol* 74(7): 990–999.

Johnson, K. (1963). "A study of the dimensional changes occuring in the maxilla after tooth extraction. Part 1: Normal healing." *Aust Dent J* 8: 428–434.

Johnson, K. (1969). "A study of the dimensional changes occurring in the maxilla following closed face immediate denture treatment." *Aust Dent J* 14(6): 370–376.

Lekovic, V., E. B. Kenney, et al. (1997). "A bone regenerative approach to alveolar ridge maintenance following tooth extraction: Report of 10 cases." *J Periodontol* 68(6): 563–570.

Schropp, L., A. Wenzel, et al. (2003). "Bone healing and soft tissue contour changes following single-tooth extraction: A clinical and radiographic 12-month prospective study." *Int J Periodontics Restorative Dent* 23(4): 313–323.

Van der Weijden, F., F. Dell'Acqua, et al. (2009). "Alveolar bone dimensional changes of post-extraction sockets in humans: A systematic review." *J Clin Periodontol* 36(12): 1048–1058.

Methods of Extraction 6

Implant dentistry has not only revolutionized the ability to treat fully and partially edentulous patients; it has also enlightened the clinician with the virtues of bone preservation following tooth extraction. The ability to treat a site with a dental implant begins with one's decision on the method of tooth extraction. This is of critical importance, especially when an immediate implant placement protocol is desired, given that this modality of treatment demands that the implant be primarily stable upon insertion via the lateral walls of the socket or virgin bone available at the apex (Lazzara 1989). Quite often, iatrogenic trauma to the surrounding hard tissues of the socket may prevent primary stability from being obtained and the immediate procedure will need to be aborted, with an early or delayed approach to placement required (Figure 6.1) (Chen, Wilson, et al. 2004).

Despite various claims of certain extraction techniques as being "atraumatic," all extraction methods impose some level of hard and/or soft

tissue trauma. Every tooth one encounters for extraction offers unique challenges when immediate implant placement is to follow (Fugazzotto 2002; Fugazzotto 2006; Fugazzotto 2008). This chapter provides insight into the various methods, instruments, and techniques available to the clinician to best preserve the

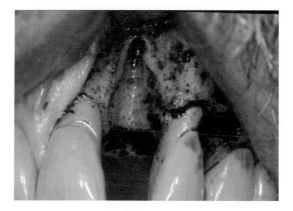

Figure 6.1 Buccal view of iatrogenic trauma with tooth extraction.

Surgical Essentials of Immediate Implant Dentistry, First Edition. Jay R. Beagle.
© 2013 John Wiley & Sons, Inc. Published 2013 by John Wiley & Sons, Inc.

hard and soft tissues, in the face of the unique challenges each extraction site presents.

DENTAL FORCEPS

It is probably correct to assume that the extraction of teeth, due to caries or fracture, dates back to the beginning of mankind. The use of an extraction forceps was described by Aristotle (384–322 BC) as two levers acting in contrary sense with a single fulcrum (Ring 1985). Forceps today have evolved to a variety of shapes and sizes, often specific to both deciduous and permanent teeth in the maxilla or mandible (Figure 6.2). These devices are designed to grip the affected tooth by the anatomic crown, remaining root structure, or furcation region, and provide the clinician with a greater mechanical advantage to remove the tooth. One must keep in mind the tooth is maintained in the socket via the periodontal ligament. Therefore, the objective in the extraction of teeth is to separate or sever the periodontal ligament from the tooth, most often using a rotation movement applied to the long axis of the root (Leonard 2002). Quite often, practitioners view the purpose of the dental forceps as to enable the rocking of the tooth in a buccal-lingual direction in an effort to expand the alveolar process for the delivery of the tooth.

When this protocol is followed, it becomes a contest between the integrity of the root of the tooth and the integrity of the buccal bone plate. If the bone is stronger than the root, then the root fractures. If the root is stronger than the bone, then a resulting dehiscence will arise with the fractured buccal plate. In light of the desire to preserve the intact alveolus for the purpose of immediate implant placement, the forceps' role should be limited to assisting in the stretching and severing of the periodontal ligament, and to delivery of the tooth or root. This implies that all teeth should be treated as single roots and therefore multi-rooted teeth should be sectioned prior to applying the site-

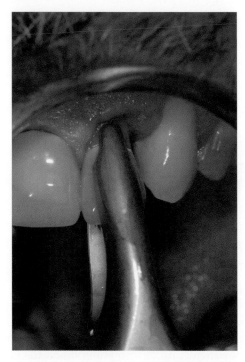

Figure 6.2   Illustration of anatomical forceps for a maxillary incisor.

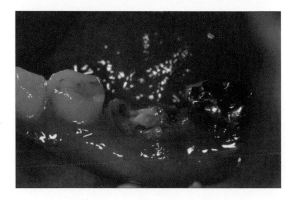

Figure 6.3   Buccal pre-op view of tooth #19.

appropriate forceps (Figures 6.3 and 6.4). When used correctly, the forceps should generate a gradual force applied clockwise to the long axis of the root for approximately 10 seconds before reversing the force counterclockwise. In many instances, it will become necessary to narrow the coronal aspect of the crown in a

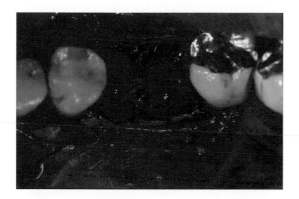

Figure 6.4 Occlusal view of #19 site following sectioning and extraction.

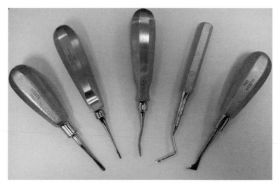

Figure 6.5 Dental elevators of various shapes and sizes.

mesial-distal direction to permit proper rotation. This exercise is repeated until the tooth loosens and is then delivered coronally to prevent fracture of the labial plate. Care should be given to observe any minute fractures of the thin buccal plate when rotating the tooth. Should this occur due to an oval-shaped root, a consideration should be made to section the root vertically using a surgical bur and handpiece to avoid further trauma.

DENTAL ELEVATORS

A simple machine is a device designed to apply or transmit force or torque. Simple machines consist of levers, inclined planes, wheels, screws, and pulleys. A dental elevator is therefore a combination of two simple machines—a lever and an inclined plane. The principle of a lever was originally described by Archimedes (circa 350 BC). The first reference to the use of a simple lever (elevator) to lift a tooth from its socket was by Abulkasim (1050–1122 AD) (Atkinson 2002). Much like dental forceps, elevators are available in a variety of shapes and sizes to apply a vertical or lateral force to a tooth root (Figure 6.5). When used with a vertical force, the wedge shape of an elevator provides the clinician a greater mechanical advantage to initiate the luxation of a tooth for

its removal when pushed along the long axis of the root surface (Misch 2008). At minimum, the width of dental elevators measures 1.5mm, while the space of the periodontal ligament ranges from 0.1mm to 0.3mm. Using an elevator for the purposes of initially luxating a tooth along its long axis most frequently results in crushing the thin interproximal bone along the mesial and/or distal, and in the esthetic zone, may affect the ability to develop an ideal papilla form. Another concern when using elevators to luxate teeth along the long axis is the possibility of increasing the mesial distal width of the socket, preventing an immediate implant from engaging the lateral walls of the site for primary stability.

Designated as a pure lever, a dental elevator can lift a tooth from its socket, via stretching and severing the periodontal ligament. The fulcrum used in this exercise is either the boney margin adjacent to the tooth or the crown/root of an adjacent tooth. In either instance, care must be given when the lever action is applied to either tissue. Injudicious force to an adjacent tooth may cause iatrogenic damage in the form of tooth fracture, restoration fracture, tooth loosening, or tooth loss. Again, as was discussed with elevators used as luxation devices along the long axis of the tooth, a dental elevator used to lift a tooth as a lever machine can crush the interproximal bone margin in an apical direction, resulting in the inability to develop an appropriate papilla form, especially in the esthetic zone.

With regards to site preparation for the immediate placement of dental implants, dental elevators present a significant liability to the bone crest and lateral socket walls. Other than applying a force to assist in separating a nearly sectioned tooth root, their role in immediate implant placement should be limited.

DENTAL LUXATORS AND PERIOTOMES

Falling into a similar category of dental instruments, luxators and periotomes are designed to severe the periodontal ligament to allow removal of the root with dental forceps or hemostats. Luxators and periotomes are both hand instruments, with periotomes consisting of a thin, somewhat flexible "blade" and the luxator having a somewhat large and pointed tip with a ridged shank. It is this more robust design that permits a luxator to be used in conjunction with a surgical mallet when used along the long axis of a tooth. Both luxators and periotomes are available in different shapes and designs to allow the clinician access to the circumference of the tooth exposed at the osseous crest.

Before applying a luxator or periotome, it is beneficial to horizontally section the clinical crown from the tooth to be extracted to provide access to the entire root perimeter. Quite often, a 15 blade can be used to initiate penetration into the periodontal ligament space before inserting the tip of the luxator or periotome. Vertical force is then applied from the instrument to the long axis of the tooth, severing the periodontal ligament (Quayle 1990). As force is applied, the blade of the instrument is rocked parallel to the root within the periodontal ligament using a pendulum motion, with the tip as a center of rotation. Frequently, this exercise is needed only along the mesial and

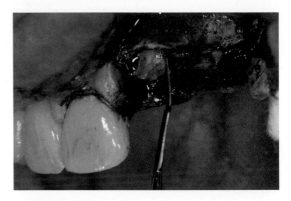

Figure 6.6   Illustration of a periotome when treating tooth #10.

distal of a root, and rarely more than two-thirds of the root length to permit removal with a forceps as previously described (Figure 6.6). Occasionally, these instruments are used along the buccal and lingual root surfaces, but care must be given to situations where the buccal plate is quite thin (<1 mm) to prevent the development of a dehiscence or fenestration defect. The clinician must also be aware of maintenance issues with both instruments. Luxators will require occasional sharpening, while the blades of periotomes may fracture under heavy force or long-term use (Leonard 2002).

VERTICAL ROOT DISTRACTORS

Severe caries or root fractures may limit one's access and instrumentation to easily extract roots with forceps, elevators, luxators, or periotomes. Quite often, mucoperiosteal flaps and resectioning of bone is required when removing teeth that are significantly destroyed in an effort to access their root surface, as a reduction in bone height as a consequence of osseous resection will influence the soft tissue contours adjacent to the implant restoration. Vertical root distractors permit the extraction of roots regardless of the ability to access the

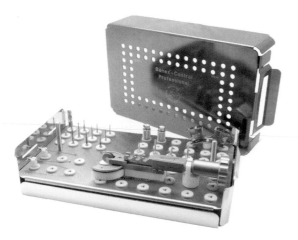

Figure 6.7 Benex control device. Reprinted with permission from Meisinger USA.

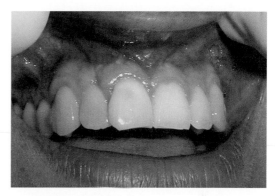

Figure 6.8 Pre-treatment view of tooth #9. Courtesy of A-Titan Instruments.

surrounding root surface. These devices use a combination of wheels, pulleys, and lever arm physics to stretch and sever the periodontal ligament and deliver the extracted root (Figure 6.7). After horizontally sectioning the clinical crown, a post space is created using a bur within the long axis of the tooth. A post of appropriate length is then selected and screwed into the created space. A special perforated impression tray to be used as a fulcrum is then filled with impression material and positioned over the post and adjacent tooth. The pulley and cable device is attached to the post, permitting the wheel to be rotated, placing tension on the cable/post device. Using a vertical force vector, the pdl of the root gradually stretches and severs, allowing for the root to be retrieved (Figures 6.8–6.15).

With no peer-reviewed studies available for review, it appears the vertical root distraction devices may offer an opportunity for an extraction with low trauma, regardless of tooth condition and elevation of mucoperiosteal flaps. This may be of significance for the immediate implant placement protocol in the esthetic zone, or sites where socket dimensions offer a challenge to obtain primary mechanical stability. The limiting factors for this device

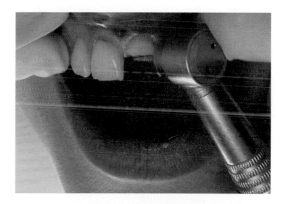

Figure 6.9 Shortening of the clinical crown of tooth #9. Courtesy of A-Titan Instruments.

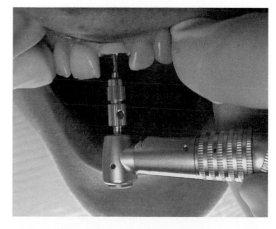

Figure 6.10 Prepping post space for tooth #9. Courtesy of A-Titan Instruments.

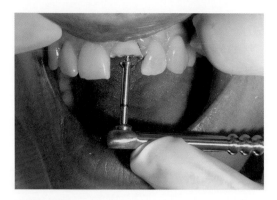

Figure 6.11   Placing post into tooth #9. Courtesy of A-Titan Instruments.

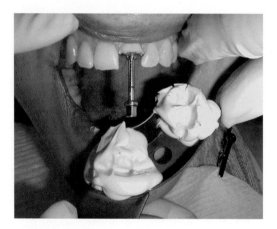

Figure 6.12   Placement of distractor tray for tooth #9. Courtesy of A-Titan Instruments.

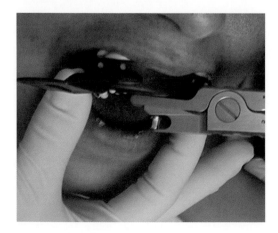

Figure 6.13   Distractor and tray in place. Courtesy of A-Titan Instruments.

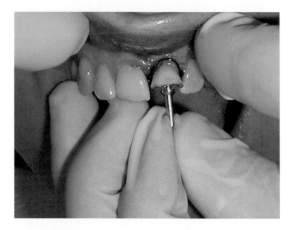

Figure 6.14   Removal of tooth #9 following distraction. Courtesy of A-Titan Instruments.

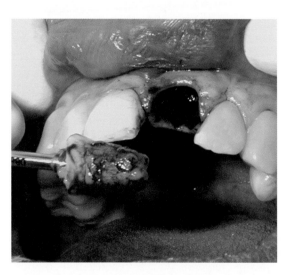

Figure 6.15   Note presentation of the soft tissue adjacent to teeth #8 and #10. Courtesy of A-Titan Instruments.

include roots that are severely dilacerated, lack of adjacent teeth, and access to posterior sites.

PIEZO SURGERY

Piezo surgery was developed by Vercellotti as a surgical method for dental osteoplasty and ostectomy (Vercellotti 2004). Using piezoelectric ultrasonic vibrations at a frequency of 29 kHz and a

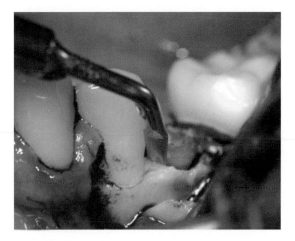

Figure 6.16 Piezo surgery being used to remove tooth #20.

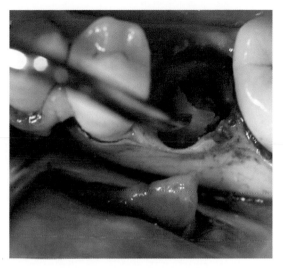

Figure 6.17 Note the presentation of the socket wall architecture following the use of piezo surgery.

range of 60/200 Hz, the resulting microvibrations permit a selective cut of only mineralized tissue without trauma to soft tissues. Through the benefit of cavitation, a virtual blood-free surgical site is possible when compared to alternative methods of bone resection using a diamond or carbide bur. Piezo surgery has demonstrated a more favorable osseous healing response and better bone remodeling as shown histologically, and it offers a variety of other dental applications involving osseous surgery such as crown lengthening, root planing, autogenous bone harvesting, periapical surgery, distraction osteogenesis, sinus window preparations, implant site osteotomies, and dental extractions (Figures 6.16 and 6.17) (Vercellotti, Nevins, et al. 2005).

A number of companies manufacture piezo surgical units for dental procedures and have a wide variety of cutting tips that permit the clinician to perform the intended procedure. Periotome-style inserts are available for use with the piezo surgical units to sever the periodontal ligament and remove minimal hard tissue lining the socket walls. Using the manufacturer's recommended power/water settings for the inserts, the tip/edge is positioned adjacent to the root surface and gently guided into the periodontal ligament space using the same movements as described with

the periotome. Again, horizontal sectioning of the clinical crown is advantageous to permit visibility of the entire root circumference, prior to using the piezo surgical device. Light pressure and constant movement of the tip in a lateral and apical direction is required to advance the leading edge of the insert parallel to the long axis of the root. Once two-thirds of the length of mesial and distal root have been treated, a forceps retrieval of the root becomes possible. If the root does not have enough root surface exposed coronal to the osseous crest to permit engagement of the forceps beaks, then the root should be vertically sectioned and the individual pieces elevated out of the socket.

Often, ankylosed teeth are recommended for extraction with the desire for immediate implant placement. Traditional methods of ankylosed tooth removal frequently result in significant trauma to the bone in these situations and may affect the outcome of the final soft tissue profile. Several peer-reviewed publications have shown the benefit and ease with which piezo surgery handles this problematic situation, without adversely affecting the surrounding hard and soft tissues (Fugazzotto 2008; Blus and Szmukler-Moncler 2010).

References

Atkinson, H. F. (2002). "Some early dental extraction instruments including the pelican, bird or axe?" *Aust Dent J* 47(2): 90–93.

Blus, C., and S. Szmukler-Moncler (2010). "Atraumatic tooth extraction and immediate implant placement with piezosurgery: Evaluation of 40 sites after at least 1 year of loading." *Int J Periodontics Restorative Dent* 30(4): 355–363.

Chen, S. T., T. G. Wilson, Jr., et al. (2004). "Immediate or early placement of implants following tooth extraction: Review of biologic basis, clinical procedures, and outcomes." *Int J Oral Maxillofac Implants* 19 Suppl: 12–25.

Fugazzotto, P. A. (2008). "Implant placement at the time of mandibular molar extraction: Description of technique and preliminary results of 341 cases." *J Periodontol* 79(4): 737–747.

Fugazzotto, P. A. (2006). "Implant placement at the time of maxillary molar extraction: Technique and report of preliminary results of 83 sites." *J Periodontol* 77(2): 302–309.

Fugazzotto, P. A. (2002). "Implant placement in maxillary first premolar fresh extraction sockets: Description of technique and report of preliminary results." *J Periodontol* 73(6): 669–674.

Lazzara, R. J. (1989). "Immediate implant placement into extraction sites: Surgical and restorative advantages." *Int J Periodontics Restorative Dent* 9(5): 332–343.

Leonard, M. (2002). "Extraction of teeth: Some general observations." *Dentistry Today* (August).

Misch, C. (2008). Contemporary Implant Dentistry, 3rd ed. St. Louis: Mosby.

Quayle, A. A. (1990). "Atraumatic removal of teeth and root fragments in dental implantology." *Int J Oral Maxillofac Implants* 5(3): 293–296.

Ring, M. (1985). *Dentistry: An Illustrated History.* New York: Harry N. Abrams.

Vercellotti, T. (2004). "Technological characteristics and clinical indications of piezoelectric bone surgery." *Minerva Stomatol* 53(5): 207–214.

Vercellotti, T., M. L. Nevins, et al. (2005). "Osseous response following resective therapy with piezosurgery." *Int J Periodontics Restorative Dent* 25(6): 543–549.

Surgical Protocol

7

The placement of an immediate dental implant offers unique challenges to the surgeon compared to placement at other time points following tooth extraction. These issues have been addressed by numerous authors over the years, yielding a "basic" surgical protocol with universally accepted pre-requisites for successful osseointegration (Gelb 1993; Lazzara 1993; Schwartz-Arad and Chaushu 1997; Chen, Wilson, et al. 2004; Chen, Beagle, et al. 2009). Regardless of the site being treated, the morphology of the extraction socket is essential in the placement of an immediate dental implant and affects the clinician's choice of flap designs, implant size selection, achievement of primary stability, necessity for hard tissue grafting, and whether to submerge or non-submerge the implant during healing. The violation of these basic tenets for immediate implant placement may result in a significant complication, and the surgeon may find the site best treated using a different timetable following tooth extraction. This chapter will focus on the salient aspects of

the immediate placement technique and offer special considerations for sites requiring unique challenges.

PRE-SURGICAL PREPARATION

No variation from the standard protocol for non-immediate placement is instituted pre-surgically. The patient should begin with a broad-spectrum antibiotic 24 hours prior to treatment and continue for a period of 10 days post-surgery. One hour prior to treatment, the patient should be given an anti-sialagogue to reduce salivary secretions, as well as a non-steroidal anti-inflammatory. Prior to delivering a local anesthetic to the site, the patient should rinse with chlorhexidine for 30 seconds and the extraoral tissues should be scrubbed and prepped from nose to chin using an antimicrobial scrub such as Betadine. In situations in which the patient is quite anxious, or when the

Surgical Essentials of Immediate Implant Dentistry, First Edition. Jay R. Beagle.
© 2013 John Wiley & Sons, Inc. Published 2013 by John Wiley & Sons, Inc.

surgical procedure is to be lengthy, the use of an oral, IM, or IV sedation should be considered. Local anesthesia using lidocaine 2% in an epinephrine concentration of 1:100,000 or 1:50,000 should be utilized for those patients having no allergies to the medication. Delivery of the anesthesia should be via infiltration to the surgical area. Block style anesthesia methods should be avoided, especially in the mandibular posterior sextants.

INCISION DESIGNS

The majority of sites treated will benefit from a full-thickness flap design as opposed to a flapless technique (Figures 7.1–7.6). Flapless techniques should only be employed when there is a favorable zone of attached gingiva, there are low esthetic demands, and the site has been assessed radiographically with a cone beam CT scan indicating favorable clinical conditions such as intact, thick facial boney walls. Anterior and posterior sites can be treated with minimal horizontal flap extension that can often be limited to only the tooth being replaced by the implant. It is generally necessary to utilize a vertical releasing incision into the mesial or distal papilla to gain access to the site and inspect the buccal plate for any dehiscence or fenestration defects. Bilateral vertical releasing incisions are suggested in sites where flap advancement is desired for a submerged or semi-submerged healing approach. This is often the case in the esthetic zone to allow for overcontouring of the buccal profile using soft and/or hard tissue grafting.

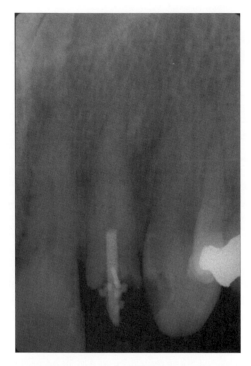

Figure 7.2   Pre-op radiograph of tooth #10.

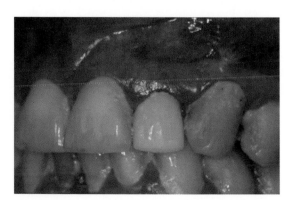

Figure 7.1   Pre-op buccal view of tooth #10 placement for extraction and immediate implant placement.

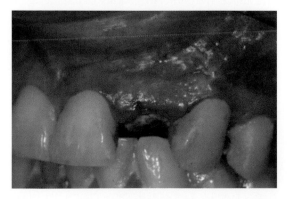

Figure 7.3   Pre-op of tooth #10 with crown removed.

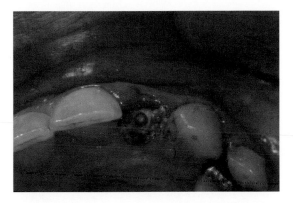

Figure 7.4 Pre-op occlusal view of tooth #10.

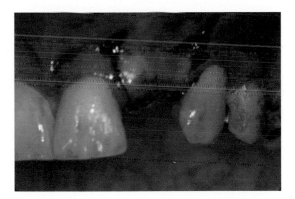

Figure 7.5 Initial incision design for full-thickness flap elevation.

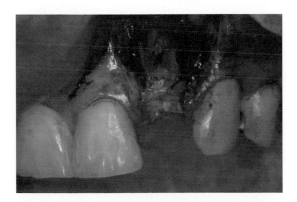

Figure 7.6 Full-thickness buccal flap elevation illustrating root surface fenestration.

TOOTH EXTRACTION

One of the keys to successful immediate implant placement is to minimize trauma to the site during the extraction process (Figures 7.7 and 7.8). In a previous chapter, a variety of methods were discussed regarding extraction protocols and instrumentation. All teeth should be viewed as either a single root or multiple single roots, as in the case of maxillary first premolars and all molars. As such, multi-rooted teeth should be sectioned into separate roots prior to removal in an effort to avoid trauma to the hard tissues. No universal method of tooth removal is suitable for all teeth, and the clinician must rely upon his or her level of experience when dealing with particularly difficult sites. Quite often, the extraction phase of the treatment may require the greatest percentage

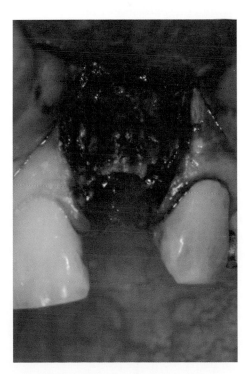

Figure 7.7 Buccal view of tooth #10 site following extraction with a periotome.

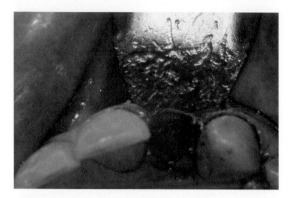

Figure 7.8   Occlusal view of tooth #10 site following extraction with a periotome.

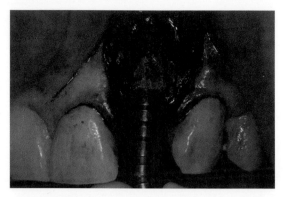

Figure 7.9   Try-in of 2.2 mm depth gauge before osteotomy.

of treatment time to preserve the site for immediate implant placement.

SITE PREPARATION

Following the extraction, the site should be thoroughly degranulated and all remnants of fibers and soft tissues removed with curettes and/or low-speed rotary instrumentation using a round diamond bur, with copious chilled irrigation (Figures 7.9–7.12). Using a series of depth gauges of various diameters, the site should be inspected and a determination made as to whether the implant can be successfully positioned into an ideal prosthetic relationship with primary mechanical stability. The morphology of the extractions socket will give the clinician guidance as to the length and diameter of implant to be chosen to obtain primary mechanical stability. In almost all situations, there will be both a vertical and horizontal defect between the implant and socket walls following placement.

The preparation of the osteotomy should follow the sequence of round burs, pilot drills, twist drills, and profile drills as recommended by the given manufacturers. All mechanical preparations should be performed using handpiece speeds of <800 RPM with copious irrigation using chilled saline. For maxillary incisors

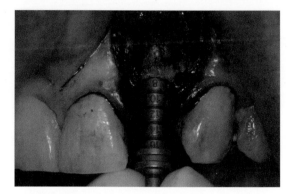

Figure 7.10   Try-in of 2.8 mm depth gauge before osteotomy.

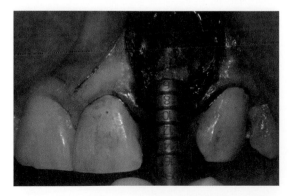

Figure 7.11   Try-in of 3.5 mm depth gauge before osteotomy.

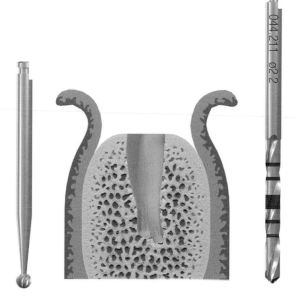

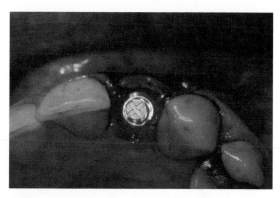

Figure 7.13 Occlusal view of immediate implant placement for tooth #10.

Figure 7.12 Diagram of round bur/pilot drill penetration location into extraction socket. Images courtesy of Straumann USA, LLC, its parents, affiliates or subsidiaries. © Straumann USA LLC, all rights reserved.

and position the restorative platform 2–4 mm from the cervical of the planned restoration (Buser, Martin, et al. 2004). The use of a surgical guide generated from a laboratory wax-up can greatly help in the 3-D positioning of the implant at the time of surgical preparation.

IMPLANT SELECTION

and maxillary cuspids, it is paramount to direct the preparation along the palatal wall of the extraction socket and initially engages bone 2–3 mm coronal to the root apex. If this guideline is not followed, the implant will be positioned too close to the labial plate, potentially resulting in a poor esthetic outcome due to loss of crestal bone and associated marginal tissue recession. Proper positioning of immediate implants in the maxillary second premolar and the mandibular incisors, cuspids, and premolars directs the initial preparation toward the root apex. For multi-rooted teeth, it is desirable to initiate the osteotomy preparation into the inter-root septum. In all instances, the axial orientation of the preparation should allow for a direct screw-retained restoration with the access located in the cingulum of anterior teeth or central fossae of posterior teeth, or alternatively, a cemented restoration using a stock abutment without modifications.

The depth of the osteotomy should allow for primary mechanical stability to be achieved

Care should be taken to avoid the placement of wide diameter or wide platform implants in esthetic zone sites (Figure 7.13). In many instances, implants exceeding the morphology of the socket will result in complications arising as mucosal recession resulting from the restorative platform being positioned too far facially (Chen, Darby, et al. 2007). This cannot be easily corrected. It is therefore suggested that maxillary central incisors and cuspids and premolars, as well as mandibular cuspids and premolars, be treated with implants having a diameter of approximately 4 mm, while maxillary lateral incisors and mandibular incisors not exceed 3.5 mm in diameter. All molars are best treated using an implant design having a wide restorative platform. Selection of an implant with a threaded profile and roughened surface offers greater predictability for osseointegration and initial stability. This is particularly relevant when the site may be influenced by external factors such as a removable prosthesis, tongue, foods, and immediate fixed provisionalization. When using an implant design having a reduced thread radius, it is desirable to slightly under-prepare the diameter of the osteotomy site by 0.2–0.5 mm in an effort to achieve primary stability. Tapered-design implants are helpful in reducing the HDD present at a site (Wilson, Schenk, et al. 1998) but should not be employed as an effort to achieve primary stability at the osseous crest, as this could lead to compression necrosis and loss of crestal bone support and height. Implant designs having either a vertical or horizontal platform shift should be chosen with the immediate placement protocol especially in the anterior zone to aid in the control of the eventual abutment/crown cement line interface, as well as eliminating the negative influence of a microgap at the osseous crest (Cochran, Hermann, et al. 1997; Hartman and Cochran 2004; Wennstrom, Ekestubbe, et al. 2005; Broggini, McManus, et al. 2006; Lazzara and Porter 2006; Zipprich, Weigl, et al. 2007; Jung, Jones, et al. 2008).

HEALING ABUTMENTS

The selection of healing abutments or closure screws should be based upon a variety of factors at the time of surgery. Should an implant be deemed to have minimal mechanical stability, a closure screw or short healing abutment should be chosen to reduce external influences from traumatizing the site and preventing osseointegration regardless of whether the site is anterior or posterior.

An extended healing abutment is desired especially in the esthetic zone to assist in the support of a coronally positioned flap. Quite often, a hard or soft tissue graft can be positioned between the healing abutment and flap to further enhance the esthetic outcome. Alternatively, a custom healing abutment can be employed when the flap is repositioned at the pre-operative gingival level. Custom healing abutments have the unique ability to more closely represent the

subgingival profile of the extracted tooth and accurately support the soft tissues without the aid of a hard or soft tissue graft. Both extended healing abutments and custom healing abutments are used most often with the semi-submerged or non-submerged flap closure technique.

HDD/VDD

Invariably, the placement of an immediate dental implant often results in either a horizontal (HDD) or vertical (VDD) gap between the implant surface and alveolar socket (Figures 7.14–7.15). Much attention has been given in the literature regarding the need to obturate this gap with a hard tissue graft or leave the gap untreated but covered with the mucoperiosteal flap. Most authors agree that should the HDD be measured as <2 mm, no augmentation of the defect is required and success will be dependent upon maintaining bone viability; stabilization of the blood clot; and prevention of inflammation, soft tissue collapse, and epithelial downgrowth (Gher, Quintero, et al. 1994; Hammerle, Chiantella, et al. 1998; Cornelini, Scarano, et al. 2000; Paolantonio, Dolci, et al. 2001; Covani, Bortolaia, et al. 2004). However, there are many situations that arise when the defects are considered quite complex and therefore benefit from hard tissue grafting as well as the use of barrier membranes. Many grafting and membrane materials have been discussed in the literature regarding the treatment of defects associated with immediate placement techniques, with all showing favorable clinical outcomes. One exception to this is the use of ePTFE membranes, which can become prematurely exposed and subsequently infected (Gher, Quintero, et al. 1994; van Steenberghe, Callens, et al. 2000), and as such, the clinician may best select any number of resorbable membranes offered today. A favorite sandwich technique employed by many is to place a particulate autogenous bone graft adjacent to the exposed implant surface and veneer a layer

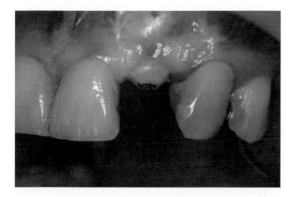

Figure 7.23 Buccal view following placement of custom healing abutment.

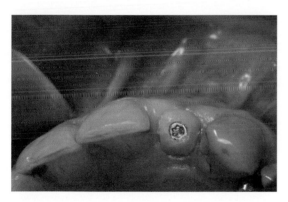

Figure 7.24 Occlusal view following placement of custom healing abutment.

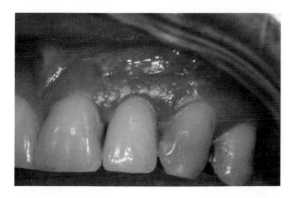

Figure 7.25 Final restoration of immediate implant replacing tooth #10.

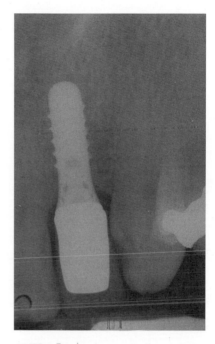

Figure 7.26 Final radiograph of immediate implant replacing tooth #10.

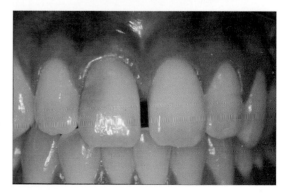

Figure 7.27 Pre-op buccal view of tooth #8 requiring immediate implant placement due to resorption of the crown/root.

would apply to severely compromised sites that may have reduced initial stability and/or the need for significant hard tissue grafting. In these circumstances, restorative treatment may be delayed until 16–20 weeks post-surgery (Figures 7.27–7.54).

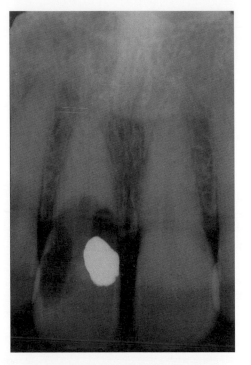

Figure 7.28 Pre-op radiograph of tooth #8.

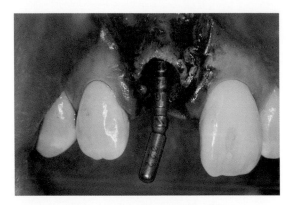

Figure 7.31 Buccal view of 2.2 depth gauge following the use of the 2.2 mm pilot drill.

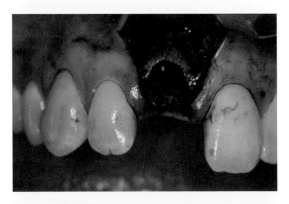

Figure 7.29 Full-thickness flap illustrating incision design.

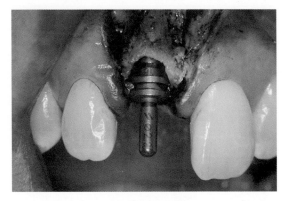

Figure 7.32 Buccal view of the 2.8 mm depth gauge following the use of the 2.8 mm twist drill.

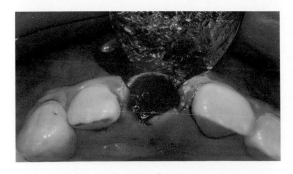

Figure 7.30 Occlusal view of thin labial bone plate.

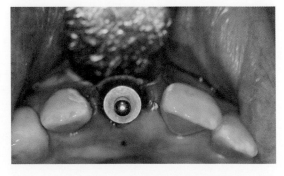

Figure 7.33 Occlusal view of the 2.8 mm depth gauge following the use of the 2.8 mm twist drill.

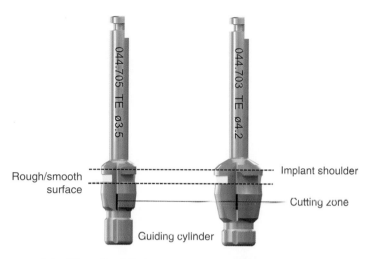

Figure 7.34 Diagram of the TE profile drill. Images courtesy of Straumann USA, LLC, its parents, affiliates or subsidiaries. © Straumann USA LLC, all rights reserved.

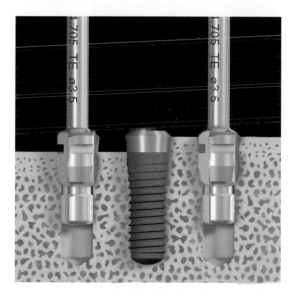

Figure 7.35 Diagram of the relationship of the TE profile drill to the posterior of the TE implant when inserted into the osteotomy. Images courtesy of Straumann USA, LLC, its parents, affiliates or subsidiaries. © Straumann USA LLC, all rights reserved.

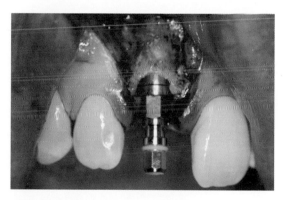

Figure 7.36 Buccal view of immediate implant insertion for tooth #8.

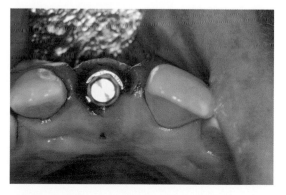

Figure 7.37 Occlusal view of immediate implant insertion for tooth #8.

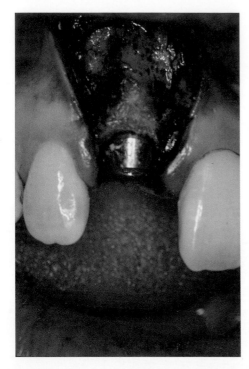

Figure 7.38   Buccal view showing the placement of a beveled healing abutment.

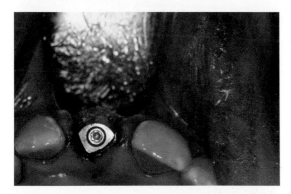

Figure 7.39   Occlusal view of the immediate implant placement for tooth #8 and addition of an autogenous bone graft into the vertical/horizontal defect between the implant and labial plate.

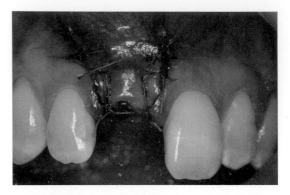

Figure 7.40   Buccal view of semi-submerged flap closure.

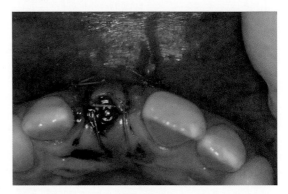

Figure 7.41   Occlusal view of semi-submerged flap closure.

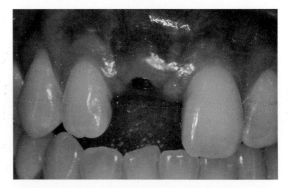

Figure 7.42   Buccal view of 12-week post-op.

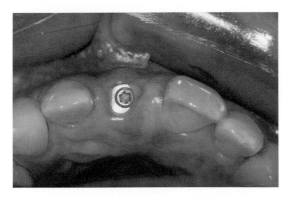

Figure 7.43 Occlusal view of 12-week post-op.

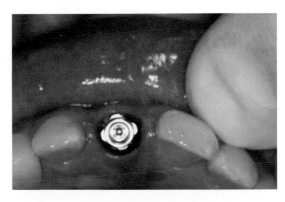

Figure 7.46 Occlusal view of the provisionalization coping.

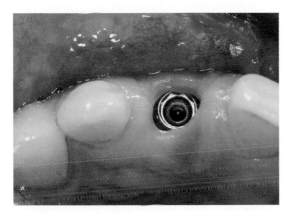

Figure 7.44 Occlusal view of 12-week post-op with healing abutment removed.

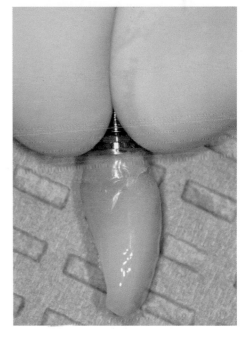

Figure 7.47 Sagital view of fabrication of fixed acrylic provisional crown.

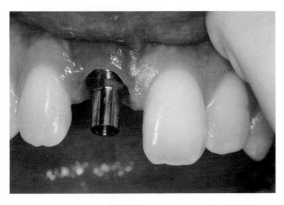

Figure 7.45 Buccal view of the provisionalization coping.

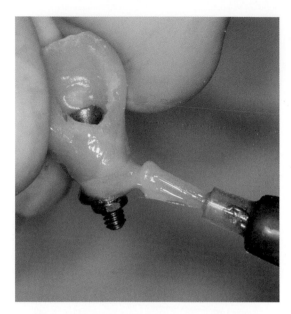

Figure 7.48 Margination of fixed acrylic provisional crown.

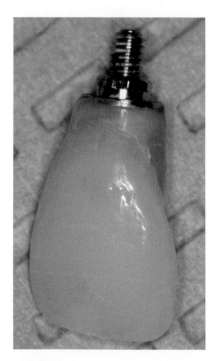

Figure 7.49 Buccal view of fixed acrylic provisional crown.

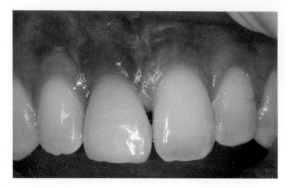

Figure 7.50 Buccal view of fixed provisional crown.

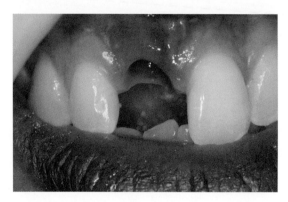

Figure 7.51 Buccal view of tissue conditioning with fixed provisional crown.

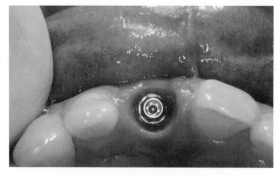

Figure 7.52 Occlusal view of tissue conditioning with fixed provisional crown.

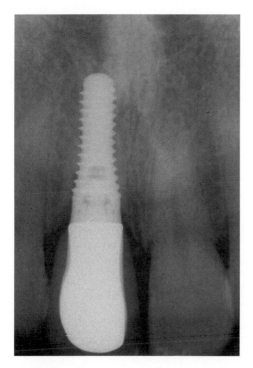

Figure 7.53 Final radiograph of immediate implant placement for tooth #8.

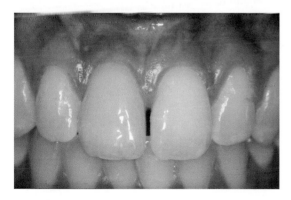

Figure 7.54 Final restoration for immediate implant placed replacing tooth #8.

References

Beagle, J. R. (2006). "The immediate placement of endosseous dental implants in fresh extraction sites." *Dent Clin North Am* 50(3): 375–389, vi.

Becker, C. M., T. G. Wilson, Jr., et al. (2011). "Minimum criteria for immediate provisionalization of single-tooth dental implants in extraction sites: A 1-year retrospective study of 100 consecutive cases." *J Oral Maxillofac Surg* 69(2): 491–497.

Broggini, N., L. M. McManus, et al. (2006). "Peri-implant inflammation defined by the implant-abutment interface." *J Dent Res* 85(5): 473–478.

Buser, D., W. Martin, et al. (2004). "Optimizing esthetics for implant restorations in the anterior maxilla: Anatomic and surgical considerations." *Int J Oral Maxillofac Implants* 19 Suppl: 43–61.

Chen, S. T., J. Beagle, et al. (2009). "Consensus statements and recommended clinical procedures regarding surgical techniques." *Int J Oral Maxillofac Implants* 24 Suppl: 272–278.

Chen, S. T., I. B. Darby, et al. (2007). "A prospective clinical study of non-submerged immediate implants: Clinical outcomes and esthetic results." *Clin Oral Implants Res* 18(5): 552–562.

Chen, S. T., T. G. Wilson, Jr., et al. (2004). "Immediate or early placement of implants following tooth extraction: Review of biologic basis, clinical procedures, and outcomes." *Int J Oral Maxillofac Implants* 19 Suppl: 12–25.

Cochran, D. L., J. S. Hermann, et al. (1997). "Biologic width around titanium implants. A histometric analysis of the implanto-gingival junction around unloaded and loaded nonsubmerged implants in the canine mandible." *J Periodontol* 68(2): 186–198.

Cornelini, R., A. Scarano, et al. (2000). "Immediate one-stage postextraction implant: A human clinical and histologic case report." *Int J Oral Maxillofac Implants* 15(3): 432–437.

Covani, U., C. Bortolaia, et al. (2004). "Buccolingual crestal bone changes after immediate and delayed implant placement." *J Periodontol* 75(12): 1605–1612.

Gelb, D. A. (1993). "Immediate implant surgery: Three-year retrospective evaluation of 50 consecutive cases." *Int J Oral Maxillofac Implants* 8(4): 388–399.

Gher, M. E., G. Quintero, et al. (1994). "Combined dental implant and guided tissue regeneration therapy in humans." *Int J Periodontics Restorative Dent* 14(4): 332–347.

Hammerle, C. H., G. C. Chiantella, et al. (1998). "The effect of a deproteinized bovine bone mineral on bone regeneration around titanium dental implants." *Clin Oral Implants Res* 9(3): 151–162.

Hartman, G. A., and D. L. Cochran (2004). "Initial implant position determines the magnitude of crestal bone remodeling." *J Periodontol* 75(4): 572–577.

Jung, R. E., A. A. Jones, et al. (2008). "The influence of non-matching implant and abutment diameters on radiographic crestal bone levels in dogs." *J Periodontol* 79(2): 260–270.

Lazzara, R. J. (1993). "Effect of implant position on implant restoration design." *J Esthet Dent* 5(6): 265–269.

Lazzara, R. J., and S. S. Porter (2006). "Platform switching: A new concept in implant dentistry for controlling postrestorative crestal bone levels." *Int J Periodontics Restorative Dent* 26(1): 9–17.

Paolantonio, M., M. Dolci, et al. (2001). "Immediate implantation in fresh extraction sockets: A controlled clinical and histological study in man." *J Periodontol* 72(11): 1560–1571.

Schwartz-Arad, D., and G. Chaushu (1997). "The ways and wherefores of immediate placement of implants into fresh extraction sites: A literature review." *J Periodontol* 68(10): 915–923.

van Steenberghe, D., A. Callens, et al. (2000). "The clinical use of deproteinized bovine bone mineral on bone regeneration in conjunction with immediate implant installation." *Clin Oral Implants Res* 11(3): 210–216.

Wennstrom, J. L., A. Ekestubbe, et al. (2005). "Implant-supported single-tooth restorations: A 5-year prospective study." *J Clin Periodontol* 32(6): 567–574.

Wilson, T. G., Jr., R. Schenk, et al. (1998). "Implants placed in immediate extraction sites: A report of histologic and histometric analyses of human biopsies." *Int J Oral Maxillofac Implants* 13(3): 333–341.

Zipprich, H., P. Weigl, et al. (2007). "Micromovements at the implant-abutment interface: Measurements, causes and consequences." *Implantologie* 15: 31–46.

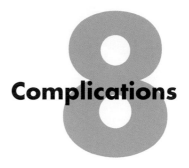

Complications

Accidents and complications are a part of clinical practice and reality in all aspects of dentistry (Annibali, Ripari, et al. 2009). A primary challenge for practitioners is to provide care to patients with the least degree of risk in an effort to achieve the highest possible functional and esthetic outcome (Dawson, Chen, et al. 2009). Patients entrust clinicians to achieve this using techniques, biomaterials, and evidence-based scientific therapy that are both time- and cost-effective. Long-term research has shown that implant dentistry, when performed with appropriate expertise and risk assessment, can yield significant success rates for replacing missing teeth; however, implant dentistry is not without risk for accidents and complications (Buser, Mericske-Stern, et al. 1997). An accident is defined as an event that occurs during a surgical or restorative procedure, while a complication is a pathologic condition that appears post-operatively. Surgical accidents can affect the soft tissues, blood vessels, nerve trunks, sinuses, and adjacent teeth. Accidents may also involve

the creation of dehiscence/fenestration defects; fractured, ingested, or inhaled instruments; and overpreparation of the osteotomy leading to the lack of primary stability (Figure 8.1). Surgical complications may result in mucosal disturbances, loss of osseointegration, technical challenges related to the restoration process, and short-/long-term esthetic and phonetic outcomes (Figure 8.2) (Adell, Lekholm, et al. 1981; Balshi 1989). Early complications following a surgical procedure can result in infections, edema, ecchymosis, hematomas, emphysema, bleeding, flap dehiscences, and sensory disorders. Late complications may consist of perforations of the mucoperiosteum, maxillary sinusitis, mandibular fractures, failed osseointegration, infraboney defects, periapical implant lesion, and peri-implantitis (Figures 8.3–8.5). Clinicians who elect to perform implant surgery must be prepared to confront these various accidents and complications when they occur. Quite often, continuing education courses designed to train dentists to

---

Surgical Essentials of Immediate Implant Dentistry, First Edition. Jay R. Beagle.
© 2013 John Wiley & Sons, Inc. Published 2013 by John Wiley & Sons, Inc.

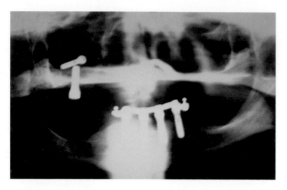

Figure 8.1   Panoramic radiograph of implant "lost" into the maxillary sinus.

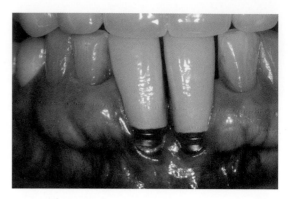

Figure 8.4   Buccal view of implants replacing teeth #24 and #25 resulting in mucositis.

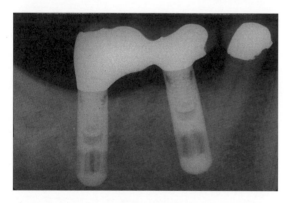

Figure 8.2   Radiograph of implant placed into the root of an adjacent premolar.

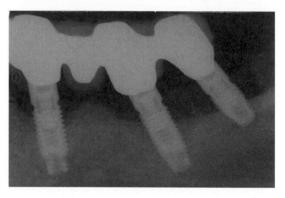

Figure 8.5   Radiograph of implants failing due to peri-implantitis.

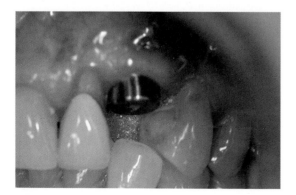

Figure 8.3   Buccal view of an implant replacing tooth #11 resulting in a fistula at the mucogingival junction.

perform implant surgery focus more on the technique aspect of the surgical procedure and spend little if any time on accidents and complications (Mattheos, Albrektsson, et al. 2009). It is for this reason that immediate implant placement should be limited to advanced and master-level surgeons, as the treatment site can frequently present with unanticipated challenges.

As with early, delayed, and late placement, the immediate placement protocol can present the clinician with the aforementioned accidents and complications. A review of the most frequently encountered issues will be described and solutions provided when possible.

NERVE AND BLOOD VESSEL INJURIES

One of the challenges with the immediate placement of dental implants into an extraction socket is obtaining primary mechanical stability. When the morphology of the site is wide, as is frequently encountered with mandibular molar and premolar sites, the osteotomy must provide the stability using intact bone apical to the root apex. It is imperative to have an accurate radiograph (periapical or CT) to locate the position of the inferior alveolar nerve and/or mental nerve. Local anesthetic should be administered as infiltration, not block, and an effort should be made to remain 2 mm coronal to the inferior alveolar nerve during the osteotomy preparation. Failure to do this may result in transient or permanent parasthesia of the mental area.

Blood vessel injuries are frequently encountered in the mandibular molar or incisor areas during the osteotomy procedure. Lingual undercuts of the mandible may not be recognized during the surgery and the lingual plate can become perforated, leading to injury to the lingual artery. This is a potential life-threatening event, and the clinician will require the expertise to address the initial hemorrhage and possible airway management concerns until the patient can be transported to the hospital.

DEHISCENCE/FENESTRATION DEFECTS

Fenestration and/or dehiscence defects are routinely encountered with the placement of immediate dental implants (Figures 8.6 and 8.7) (Zitzmann, Scharer, et al. 1999). The periodontal literature has shown that naturally occurring defects along the facial bone plate are quite common, especially with maxillary and mandibular cuspids (Rupprecht, Horning, et al. 2001). Certainly the fenestration defects are the result

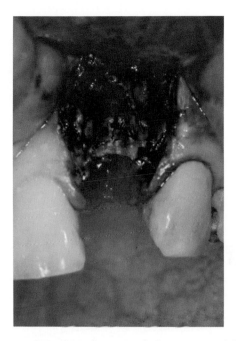

Figure 8.6 Buccal view of fenestration defect following tooth extraction.

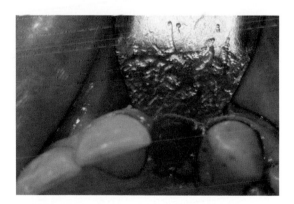

Figure 8.7 Occlusal view of the thin labial bone plate.

of a thin buccal plate and/or prominent root surface, while dehiscence defects may be the result of root/crown angulation toward the labial. Dehiscence defects may also occur due to periodontal disease, treatment of cervical caries, and the presence of a thin phenotype. Both fenestration and dehiscence defects may be the result of surgical trauma that occurs iatrogenically during the extraction or osteotomy process. When extracting a tooth with a thin labial plate, the clinician must attempt to initially use a scalpel blade or periotome to separate the root surface from the attachment fibers. The temptation to luxate the tooth using a buccal-lingual vector with a forceps should be avoided, and instead, a rotational movement as described in a previous chapter should be employed. On very difficult extractions one may wish to section the tooth to lessen the forces upon the labial plate and reduce the possibility of creating a dehiscence defect.

Fenestration defects are more commonly experienced in the maxillary arch, involving the premolars, cuspids, and incisors. Frequently the anterior maxilla has a steep labial angulation, creating an apical undercut (Figure 8.8). When preparing the osteotomy for prosthetically driven implant placement, the tip of the pilot/twist drill may penetrate the labial plate, creating a defect. One may attempt to bodily reposition the preparation toward the palatal with the subsequent diameter twist drill or simply continue but be limited with a slightly shorter implant length.

Fenestration or dehiscence defects should not result in the abortion of immediate implant placement procedure, as both can be successfully treated. Fenestration defects are most easily

addressed using either particulate autogenous bone or a bone allograft/xenograft. Ideally, a resorbable membrane can be applied over the graft before closing the flap to stabilize the graft and prevent contact with the soft tissues.

Dehiscence defects may influence the esthetic outcome of the soft tissues in relation to the implant and definitive restoration (Kan, Rungcharassaeng, et al. 2007). As a result, the clinician should use a sandwich-style graft technique to correct the dehiscence but also to support the buccal flap at the planned cervical aspect of the restoration (Buser, Wittneben, et al. 2011). The technique involves the placement of particulate autogenous bone adjacent to the implant surface followed by a veneer of xenograft. The entire graft composite is then covered with a resorbable membrane using a poncho technique and the flaps are advanced coronally (Beagle 2006).

LACK OF PRIMARY STABILITY

One of the initial keys for success with immediate implant placement is the ability to obtain primary mechanical stability (Lazzara 1989). This is accomplished by either engaging sound bone at the apical extent of the osteotomy or along the lateral walls of the preparation. Failure to achieve initial stability will lead to the inability for the implant to osseointegrate due to micro-/macro-movement. For a threaded implant design, only one or two threads engaged in bone may be enough to accomplish this goal. Many times, the clinician will know if primary stability will be difficult to achieve before the implant is placed. This may be determined radiographically or upon inspection of the extraction site morphology following tooth removal. When stability appears challenging, the clinician should exercise extreme caution when attempting to gain stability by deepening or widening the socket dimensions in relation to surrounding anatomy (inferior alveolar nerve, sinus floor, adjacent teeth). Also to be

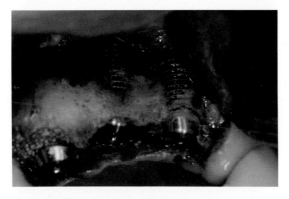

Figure 8.8   Fenestration defect encountered due to improper implant selection.

avoided is the use of a wide diameter or tapered effect implant design that might be placed in contact with a thin labial plate, resulting in compression necrosis to the bone and leading to a fenestration or dehiscence defect upon healing (Buser, Martin, et al. 2004).

MUCOSAL RECESSION

One of the strongest arguments in the literature against the immediate placement of dental implants in the esthetic zone is the greater incidence of mucosal recession following restoration. It has been reported that mucosal recession of 0.5 mm or more occurs in greater than 33% of immediately placed implants with one-fifth of the sites having 1–2 mm of recession (Chen, Beagle, et al. 2009). A number of factors can contribute to this finding, including positioning the implant shoulder too shallow or into the facial danger zone, placing the implant into a site with a thin soft or hard tissue phenotype, flapless procedures, contact of a removable provisional into the soft tissues, the fabrication of a provisional or definitive restoration having a robust convex cervical contour, and/or the use of an implant in the esthetic zone having a wide diameter/wide restorative platform (Figure 8.9) (Buser, Martin, et al. 2004; Chen, Darby, et al. 2007; Chen and Buser 2009). If

properly addressed, immediately placed dental implants can have a successful esthetic outcome without concern for mucosal recession. The clinician must utilize a restorative-driven placement protocol that routinely positions the shoulder of the implant into an ideal location, if not more palatally positioned. Tissue-level implants should position the shoulder 2 mm apical to the cervical of the planned restoration, while bone level implants should be placed 3–4 mm cervical to the planned restoration (Figures 8.10–8.15) (Buser, Chen, et al. 2008). A flapped approach is recommended to advance the soft tissues into a semi- or fully

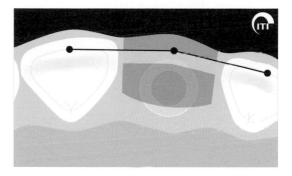

Figure 8.10 Illustration of ideal buccal-lingual positioning for tissue-level implants. From *ITI Treatment Guide*, vol. 1. Courtesy of Quintessence Publishing.

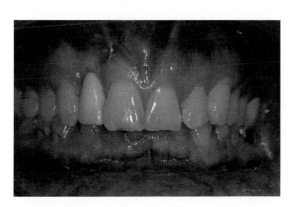

Figure 8.9 Marginal tissue recession involving tooth #7 following provisionalization.

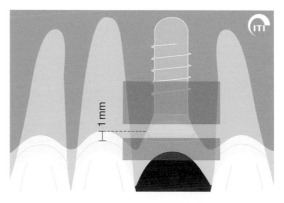

Figure 8.11 Illustration of ideal mesial-distal positioning for tissue-level implants. From *ITI Treatment Guide*, vol. 1. Courtesy of Quintessence Publishing.

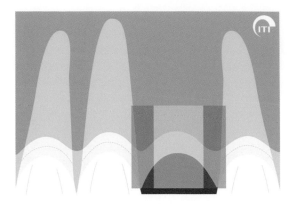

Figure 8.12 Illustration of ideal vertical relationship for implant positioning for tissue-level implants. From *ITI Treatment Guide*, vol. 1. Courtesy of Quintessence Publishing.

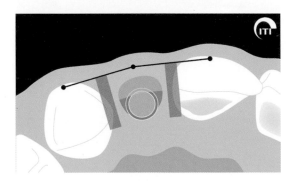

Figure 8.13 Illustration of ideal buccal-lingual positioning for bone-level implants. From *ITI Treatment Guide*, vol. 3. Courtesy of Quintessence Publishing.

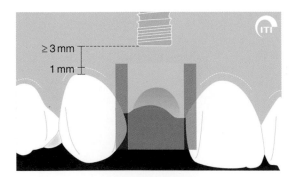

Figure 8.14 Illustration of ideal mesial-distal positioning for bone-level implants. From From *ITI Treatment Guide*, vol. 3. Courtesy of Quintessence Publishing.

submerged position, allowing the labial aspect of the implant near the crest of the ridge to be "over-engineered" with soft and/or hard tissue grafting. Access to the healing abutment following osseointegration can be made using a biopsy punch positioned toward the palatal aspect of the ridge, thereby preserving the buccal soft tissues. Finally, the lab technician and restorative dentist must ensure the cervical contour of the provisional and definitive restorations does not force the tissue into a buccal/apical location via improper over-contouring, resulting in mucosal recession (Figures 8.16–8.21) (Buser, Martin, et al. 2004).

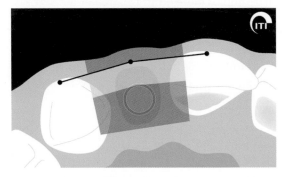

Figure 8.15 Illustration of ideal vertical relationship for positioning of bone-level implants. From *ITI Treatment Guide*, vol. 3. Courtesy of Quintessence Publishing.

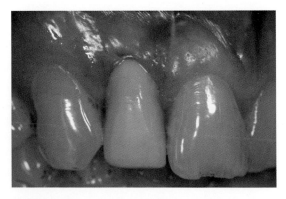

Figure 8.16 Buccal view of implant replacing tooth #7 with an overcontoured provisional restoration.

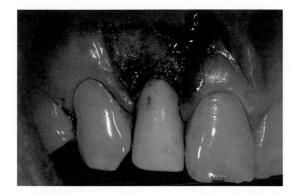

Figure 8.17 Overcontoured restoration evident with a flap elevated.

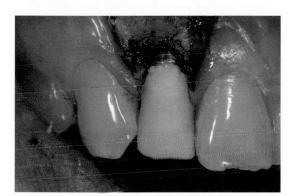

Figure 8.18 Properly contoured provisional restoration for tooth #7.

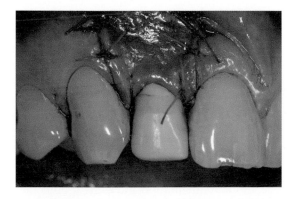

Figure 8.19 Coronally advanced flap following recontouring of provisional crown.

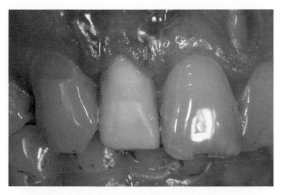

Figure 8.20 Two-week post-op of tooth #7.

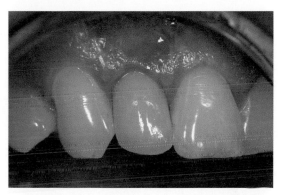

Figure 8.21 Final restoration of tooth #7.

PERI-IMPLANT DISEASE/ INFECTION

Placement of dental implants into a site with a highly scalloped soft/hard tissue architecture frequently yields deep (> 5 mm) probing depths along the interproximal and lingual aspects as opposed to the facial. This is especially true in situations involving the immediate placement of dental implants, regardless of site location, as the roughened surface of the implant is routinely placed at a level even with the buccal crestal bone. Ultimately, this deep placement protocol can create challenges for the restorative phase of treatment, and with cemented restorations may make cement removal difficult or impossible (Figures 8.22 and 8.23). For

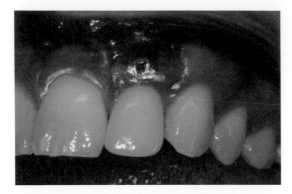

Figure 8.22 Buccal view of tooth #10 with peri-implant disease caused by retained cement.

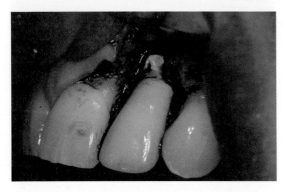

Figure 8.23 Retained cement visualized following flap elevation.

this reason, it is suggested that deeply placed immediate implants be restored with direct screw-retained restorations when possible or with a cemented crown placed onto a custom or CAD/CAM abutment. A custom or CAD/CAM abutment will allow the clinician to accurately position the cement margin 1 mm subgingival to allow for precise cement retrieval following crown delivery. Wilson (2009) has noted that peri-implant disease caused by sublingual cement occurs in 81% of all cases exhibiting mucosal inflammation, with clinical signs of this problem developing as late as 4 years post-cementation.

In the hands of an appropriately trained and experienced dental surgeon, with proper treatment planning and diagnosis, and with recognition of the unique challenges posed by both immediate implant dentistry and each patient's anatomical presentation, accidents and complications with immediate dental implants can be avoided and success achieved rivaling that of non-immediately placed dental implants. Further research and development will most certainly continue to further this trend.

References

Adell, R., U. Lekholm, et al. (1981). "A 15-year study of osseointegrated implants in the treatment of the edentulous jaw." *Int J Oral Surg* 10(6): 387–416.

Annibali, S., M. Ripari, et al. (2009). "Local accidents in dental implant surgery: Prevention and treatment." *Int J Periodontics Restorative Dent* 29(3): 325–331.

Balshi, T. J. (1989). "Preventing and resolving complications with osseointegrated implants." *Dent Clin North Am* 33(4): 821–868.

Beagle, J. R. (2006). "The immediate placement of endosseous dental implants in fresh extraction sites." *Dent Clin North Am* 50(3): 375–389, vi.

Buser, D., S. T. Chen, et al. (2008). "Early implant placement following single-tooth extraction in the esthetic zone: Biologic rationale and surgical procedures." *Int J Periodontics Restorative Dent* 28(5): 441–451.

Buser, D., W. Martin, et al. (2004). "Optimizing esthetics for implant restorations in the anterior maxilla: Anatomic and surgical considerations." *Int J Oral Maxillofac Implants* 19 Suppl: 43–61.

Buser, D., R. Mericske-Stern, et al. (1997). "Long-term evaluation of non-submerged ITI implants. Part 1: 8-year life table analysis of a prospective multi-center study with 2359 implants." *Clin Oral Implants Res* 8(3): 161–172.

Buser, D., J. Wittneben, et al. (2011). "Stability of contour augmentation and esthetic outcomes of implant-supported single crowns in the esthetic zone: 3-year results of a prospective study with early implant placement post-extraction." *J Periodontol* 82(3): 342–349.

Chen, S., and D. Buser (2009). Implant Placement in Post-Extraction Sites. Berlin: Quintessence.

Chen, S. T., J. Beagle, et al. (2009). "Consensus statements and recommended clinical procedures regarding surgical techniques." *Int J Oral Maxillofac Implants* 24 Suppl: 272–278.

Chen, S. T., I. B. Darby, et al. (2007). "A prospective clinical study of non-submerged immediate implants: Clinical outcomes and esthetic results." *Clin Oral Implants Res* 18(5): 552–562.

Dawson, A., S. Chen, et al. (2009). The SAC Classification in Implant Dentistry. Berlin: Quintessence.

Kan, J. Y., K. Rungcharassaeng, et al. (2007). "Periimplant tissue response following immediate provisional restoration of scalloped implants in the esthetic zone: A one-year pilot prospective multicenter study." *J Prosthet Dent* 97(6 Suppl): S109–118.

Lazzara, R. J. (1989). "Immediate implant placement into extraction sites: Surgical and restorative advantages." *Int J Periodontics Restorative Dent* 9(5): 332–343.

Mattheos, N., T. Albrektsson, et al. (2009). "Teaching and assessment of implant dentistry in undergraduate and postgraduate education: A European consensus." *Eur J Dent Educ* 13 Suppl 1: 11–17.

Rupprecht, R. D., G. M. Horning, et al. (2001). "Prevalence of dehiscences and fenestrations in modern American skulls." *J Periodontol* 72(6): 722–729.

Wilson, T. G., Jr. (2009). "The positive relationship between excess cement and peri-implant disease: A prospective clinical endoscopic study." *J Periodontol* 80(9): 1388–1392.

Zitzmann, N. U., P. Scharer, et al. (1999). "Factors influencing the success of GBR: Smoking, timing of implant placement, implant location, bone quality and provisional restoration." *J Clin Periodontol* 26(10): 673–682.

Index

Page numbers followed by *f* denote figures; page numbers followed by *t* denote tables.

Surgical Essentials of Immediate Implant Dentistry, First Edition. Jay R. Beagle.
© 2013 John Wiley & Sons, Inc. Published 2013 by John Wiley & Sons, Inc.